D0631853

WHAT YOUR DOCTOR
HASN'T TOLD YOU AND
THE HEALTH-STORE
CLERK DOESN'T KNOW

WHAT YOUR DOCTOR HASN'T TOLD YOU AND THE HEALTH-STORE CLERK DOESN'T KNOW

THE TRUTH ABOUT ALTERNATIVE TREATMENTS AND WHAT WORKS

EDWARD L. SCHNEIDER, M.D.

AND LEIGH ANN HIRSCHMAN

Avery | a member of Penguin Group (USA) Inc. | New York

Published by the Penguin Group

Penguin Group (USA) Inc., 375 Hudson Street, New York, New York 10014, USA • Penguin Group (Canada), 90 Eglinton Avenue East, Suite 700, Toronto, Ontario M4P 2Y3, Canada (a division of Pearson Penguin Canada Inc.) • Penguin Books Ltd, 80 Strand, London WC2R 0RL, England • Penguin Ireland, 25 St Stephen's Green, Dublin 2, Ireland (a division of Penguin Books Ltd) • Penguin Group (Australia), 250 Camberwell Road, Camberwell, Victoria 3124, Australia (a division of Pearson Australia Group Pty Ltd) • Penguin Books India Pvt Ltd, 11 Community Centre, Panchsheel Park, New Delhi–110 017, India • Penguin Group (NZ), Cnr Airborne and Rosedale Roads, Albany, Auckland 1310, New Zealand (a division of Pearson New Zealand Ltd) • Penguin Books (South Africa) (Pty) Ltd, 24 Sturdee Avenue, Rosebank, Johannesburg 2196, South Africa

Penguin Books Ltd, Registered Offices: 80 Strand, London WC2R 0RL, England

Copyright © 2006 by Edward Schneider, M.D., and Leigh Ann Hirschman
All rights reserved. No part of this book may be reproduced, scanned, or distributed in any printed or electronic form without permission. Please do not participate in or encourage piracy of copyrighted materials in violation of the authors' rights. Purchase only authorized editions.

ISBN-13: 978-1-58333-252-8

Printed in the United States of America

BOOK DESIGN BY MEIGHAN CAVANAUGH

While the authors have made every effort to provide accurate telephone numbers and Internet addresses at the time of publication, neither the publisher nor the authors assume any responsibility for errors, or for changes that occur after publication. Further, the publisher does not have any control over and does not assume any responsibility for author or third-party websites or their content.

Neither the publisher nor the authors are engaged in rendering professional advice or services to the individual reader. The ideas, procedures, and suggestions contained in this book are not intended as a substitute for consulting with your physician. All matters regarding your health require medical supervision. Neither the authors nor the publisher shall be liable or responsible for any loss or damage allegedly arising from any information or suggestion in this book. The opinions expressed in this book represent the personal views of the authors and not of the publisher.

This book is designed to help you make informed choices; it is not meant to replace formal medical treatment by a physician or other licensed health-care provider. Before using any alternative therapy, please seek appropriate medical care and carry out the treatments discussed in this book only under the guidance of a qualified professional. Pregnant and lactating women especially should *never* use alternative medicine—including but not limited to herbs, manipulative treatments, and hydrotherapy—without approval from their physicians.

This book is dedicated to my wife, Leah Buturain, who complements my life in so many ways. She embodies spirituality, poetry, beauty, and love. I am grateful to her for raising with me our four wonderful children, Samuel Raphael, Isaac Michael, Clare Gabriel Sophia, and Jakub Landau.

ACKNOWLEDGMENTS

I would like to thank my wife, Leah; her mother, Rita; and my sister, Marilyn, for inspiring me to write this book on alternative medicine. Their desire for radiant health and their respect for that which cannot be measured have sensitized me to the needs and questions of the readers I seek to serve. Truly I am blessed to have such a wonderfully supportive and creative family.

I am in deep debt to my uncle, Archie Meckler, a compassionate physician who introduced me to alternative medicine before the term even existed. Three decades after Uncle Archie inspired me to enter the healing arts, another visionary, Sandy Weiss, sponsored my first trip to China to investigate traditional Chinese medicine.

I am grateful to my distinguished colleagues: Dohwa Kim, Diana Schneider, Freddi Segal-Giddan, Joanna Davies, Glenn Stimmel, Fred Kuyt, Caleb Finch, Wayne Chen, Robert Beart, Rob Landel, and Sonia Ancoli-Israel, who reviewed the book and/or individual chapters to make sure that my information was accurate and timely. I also would like to acknowledge my friends for their support, encouragement, and input, including Warren Bennis, Gale Bensussen, Joyce Campbell, Jamie Heidegger, Miriam Hinrichs, Karen McCaffrey, Virginia Ramo, Keith Renken, Kathy Smith, Flora Thorton, Hope Warner, Teddi Winograd, Marilyn Winthrop, and Ruth Zeigler.

I could not write books without the talented USC students who have helped me compile and check all the journal articles that were used to formulate the recommendations made on these pages. Rebecca Morris, Gail Shinkawa, and Kathryn Thomas worked together as a great team to support my research.

I wish to thank Steve Sample, the president of the University of Southern California and an inspiring leader, who helped arrange the additional year of sabbatical that I used to complete this book. I would also like to recognize Michael Lombardi for establishing the Michael and Susan Lombardi/Edward L. Schneider Professorship of Gerontology at USC.

Betsy Amster is an extraordinary agent. She has skillfully guided me through the complex world of publishing. Thanks also to the crack editorial team of Megan Newman, Kristen Jennings, and Lucia Watson. These professionals have brought this book to publication with wisdom, enthusiasm, and good humor. It has been a delight to write this book with Leigh Ann Hirschman. Her writing abilities and diplomacy ensured that this book was published in a timely and professional manner.

Finally, I'd like to thank all the health providers, whether conventional or alternative, who at heart share the same goal of improving the health and well-being of humankind. This book was fueled by the desire for greater understanding between these groups.

CONTENTS

Preface: You Need This Book!   *xiii*

1 Shopping Smart for Alternative Medicine   *1*

2 Joint Pain: Improving Function,
   Easing Discomfort   *25*

3 Back on Track: Relief for Back and Neck Pain   *53*

4 Satisfying Sleep   *79*

5 Taming Depression and Anxiety   *99*

6 PMS: Natural Symptom Relief   *117*

7 Making Menopause More Comfortable   *127*

8 Revving Up Male Libido   *151*

9 **Improving Prostate Health** *161*

10 **Preventing Heart Disease and Stroke** *169*

11 **Boosting Brain Function** *199*

12 **Cancer Prevention and Treatment** *215*

13 **The Longevity Top Ten** *237*

Appendix: Take This to Your Doctor *243*

Index *259*

About the Authors *268*

PREFACE:
YOU NEED THIS BOOK!

At the hospital the other day, I saw a patient named Mr. J. My colleagues warned me that although he was obviously intelligent, Mr. J. was a difficult patient and would take up a lot of my time. Not only was he struggling under the burden of multiple health problems—including elevated blood pressure, heart disease, diabetes, insomnia, and depression—he was unhappy with the course of his medical treatment. And he let you know it. So it was with some curiosity and trepidation that I knocked on the door of the examining room where Mr. J. waited.

At the clinic where I work, we encourage patients to bring in all their prescription drugs as well as their over-the-counter medications and alternative remedies. This way we can check for potential interactions among the substances. Mr. J. had brought with him a whole shopping bag full of bottles, and I wasn't surprised to see several herbs and supplements among them. Many patients with chronic health problems turn to alternative medicine out of dissatisfaction with conventional treatment.

After adjusting Mr. J.'s blood-pressure prescription, I looked at his collection of alternative medicines. He was taking fish-oil capsules, echinacea, a high-potency multivitamin, and melatonin pills. I asked him whether the melatonin pills seemed to be helping treat his insomnia.

Mr. J.'s first reaction was surprise. I don't think many other doctors had shown interest in his alt-med stash, beyond suggesting that he dump it. Then he admitted that the melatonin wasn't working as well as he'd hoped.

I inspected the bottle and pointed out that melatonin is a short-acting substance. Half of it leaves the body less than half an hour after the pill is taken; another 25 percent departs in the next half hour. In two hours, 90 percent of the melatonin is gone. "A drug can't help you sleep if it's not in your body," I said, and I suggested that he try a delayed-release melatonin preparation that would last through the night.

Now I had his attention. I held up his echinacea pills. "There's little evidence that these do anything," I said. "And you're smart to take fish oils for your heart problems, but you don't need a combination of omega-3 and omega-6 fish oils—you need supplements with omega-3 fatty acids only, nothing more." I didn't think his choice of multivitamins was so hot, either, but I decided to leave that subject for another day.

When I left the examining room, this "difficult" patient thanked me for respecting his interest in alternative medicine and for offering some much-needed guidance. I, however, felt troubled. I'd seen too many people who, like Mr. J., suffer from a chronic health condition and are frustrated with the current medical system. By definition, most chronic disorders are incurable, and we physicians often have little to offer. The pills and treatments that *are* available often come with harsh side effects that make them unattractive, especially for long-term use. Where, then, can sufferers of arthritis, back pain, insomnia, mood disorders, heart disease, and other chronic conditions turn?

For nearly half of all adult Americans, the answer is alternative medicine, even if they're not quite sure just *which* alternatives are right for them. Unfortunately, few doctors—or alternative practitioners, for that matter—are in a position to offer objective, informed guidance about the safest and most effective alternative therapies. That's where this book steps in.

As the dean emeritus of the nation's only school of gerontology and a former deputy director of the National Institute on Aging, I am frequently invited to lecture on longevity and good health. I enjoy sharing what I've learned over the years, so I speak to groups all around the country. I talk about the latest research on aging, daily habits for longevity, and the newest information about vitamins and minerals. But no matter what I focus on, one subject *always* dominates the postlecture discussion: alternative medicine. The questions I field from audience members demonstrate the hope and uncertainty many people feel:

- Do cleansing treatments prevent cancer?
- I think I might be depressed. Could Saint-John's-wort, acupuncture, or massage help?
- Which fish oils should I take? Omega-3, omega-6, DHA, EPA, or linolenic acid? Do I risk ingesting pollutants like mercury if I take fish-oil supplements?
- I have heart disease. Should I take coenzyme Q_{10} or hawthorn?
- Will saw palmetto really shrink my prostate?
- There are hundreds of glucosamine and chondroitin products out there, alone or in combination with MSM or SAMe. How do I know which ones to buy and how much to take for arthritis pain?

Anyone who's ever asked a question like this knows what it's like to be stuck between a rock and a hard place. On one side, there are doctors who simply haven't been trained in alternative medicine. Ask them about an herbal treatment or massage therapy and you might receive a noncommittal shrug—or a blanket warning to avoid all untested products or services. On the other side are the health-store clerks and other alt-med types who don't always understand the full medical implications of the products and services they sell. I'll never forget the health-store clerk who proudly boasted to me of his "on-the-job education" . . . which consisted of nothing more than sales advice from the store's associate manager! Sadly, this scenario isn't unusual. Many health stores "educate" their salespeople in this manner; plenty of others offer their clerks health-education material that comes from biased sources, including supplement companies.

Caught between the two extremes stands the consumer. This is truly a tight spot for people who are willing to look outside conventional medicine's limited offerings for chronic pain, sleeplessness, or other common but seemingly incurable conditions—but who also want to exercise good sense and caution about health matters. Like Mr. J., you may have had the bewildering experience of wandering alone down the health-store aisles, trying to hammer out your own compromise between a doctor's medical expertise and a salesperson's attractive promises. Or perhaps you've chosen to stay at home, allowing the cloud of confusion that surrounds alternative medicine to prevent you from employing the healing methods that can help you lead a fuller life.

Even if your experience with alternative medicine has been frustrating so far, I have some good news: there are many products and treatments available that can help control those common but chronic health problems, even when conventional medicine throws up its hands. (For example, alternative medicine contributes the most reliable source of relief from back pain, a disorder that debilitates millions of Americans.) Often, these alternative approaches cost less than conventional medications and have fewer side effects. And they're not just the ones we've all read about again and again in popular magazines. I often find that even veteran alt-med consumers haven't heard about some of the best approaches for their problems.

But I'm not just a booster for the alt-med industry—no way! I'm here to help you shop smart for your health. As you may have discovered on your own, that's harder than it sounds. Plenty of popular treatments are ineffective and a waste of your money. Others can mix dangerously with other medications or health problems. Unless you've been trained in medical research and have plenty of time—not to mention the resources of medical journals and online databases—at your disposal, it's awfully hard to get sane, open-minded information about alternative medicine. That's why I wrote this book. Why should you trust me? Good question. I like it when people show a healthy dose of skepticism!

Over a career spent studying the aging process, I've seen the unlikely become mainstream. For example, who would have thought red wine and chocolate would prove to be good for you? (For more information about these tasty health foods, check out pages 175–176.) I've also seen alt-med fads come and go. For example, back in 1978, I was planning experiments with the steroid DHEA (proposed to improve immune function and glucose metabolism), alongside the great French scientist Etienne Baulieu. And like you, I've watched as conventional medicine has experienced both its triumphs, such as the 60 percent reduction in strokes through blood pressure regulation, and its dispiriting failures, including its about-face on hormone replacement therapy and the recent scare over certain pain medications. I've simply been around too long to have an ax to grind either way. I'm not employed by the pharmaceutical or alternative-medicine industries, and I don't take a penny from either one of them. As a scientist, I won't dismiss any potentially useful therapy out of hand, and I've done the painstaking research required to come to practical conclusions about alternative therapies. The result of that work is now in your hands.

How to Use This Book

This book is meant to be accessible and easy to use. It starts by helping you become a savvier customer of alternative medicine. The very first chapter lays out basic principles for understanding and evaluating alternative medicine (also known as complementary or integrative medicine). You'll get tips on shopping for supplements, discover how to evaluate scientific studies, and learn when a treatment might be worth trying even in the absence of rigorous testing. I'll also briefly survey the most popular therapeutic systems covered by the term *alternative medicine*, describing the benefits and challenges posed by each.

Chapters 2 through 12 are devoted to specific health needs. Each chapter describes a common health problem and includes a discussion of the strengths and weaknesses of the conventional treatments available, along with recommendations for lifestyle changes to treat or prevent the condition. Then comes my "Discriminating Consumer's Guide" to alternative medicine for the problem. To help you sort the wheat from the chaff, this guide analyzes the most popular alternative treatments and breaks them down into four categories:

HIGHLY RECOMMENDED: Backed by good evidence of both effectiveness and safety.

RECOMMENDED: Limited evidence of effectiveness but worth trying anyway. These therapies are usually supported by sound scientific logic and some studies of effectiveness, and are relatively safe. This category also includes a few therapies that may carry some risk but hold potential benefits for a dire and otherwise incurable condition, such as Alzheimer's disease.

ACCEPTABLE: Very little proof of effectiveness and no real scientific logic, but relatively safe to try if you like. Also included are therapies that are appropriate only under certain conditions until further evidence of safety is available.

DO NOT USE: These therapies are ineffective, unsafe, or both.

There are clear, accessible explanations of the evidence (or lack thereof) for each therapy, along with hard-to-find information about how to get the proper dosages and courses of treatment while minimizing expense and side effects.

At the end of each chapter is a fast reference called "The Complete Prescription." This guide highlights the smartest combination of conventional and alternative therapies to treat the problem under discussion.

Not everyone with an interest in alternative medicine has a chronic health disorder. Perhaps you simply wonder how to become or remain healthy, with a fresh daily supply of energy and vigor. The final chapter, "The Longevity Top Ten," provides a guide to the supplements and therapies most likely to help you stay vital for life.

When you use alternative medicines, you need to keep your doctor informed of what you're doing. (More on that in the next chapter.) To make your physician's job a little easier, I've included an appendix called "Take This to Your Doctor." As the title indicates, you can show your doctor this section, which contains citations for the medical journals I've used in compiling the "Complete Prescription" sections. If your doctor wants to check on an herb you want to take, or research the safety of chiropractic techniques, he or she can look up the appropriate reference. You can use it, too, if you'd like to learn more about these treatments for yourself.

No matter how you choose to use this book, I hope that it directs you toward relief for your chronic condition and shows you some strategies for a longer, more vibrant life. It's my intention that the advice here will fill the alarmingly wide gap between what your doctor hasn't told you and your health-store clerk doesn't know.

I

Shopping Smart for Alternative Medicine

S how me the evidence!" chortles your doctor when you inquire about alternative therapies. The strong implication here is that *no* evidence exists to support these treatments. Yet when you go to the health store, you hear a very different story. "Studies show that product X can lower blood pressure," the clerk informs you. "Scientific evidence proves that supplement Y's natural ingredients will regulate your circadian rhythms so that you can sleep more soundly."

What's going on?

When you're shopping for alternative medicine, it's not always easy to separate fact from fiction. For example: Have you heard about the long lives supposedly enjoyed by the villagers in the Caucasus Mountains of the Republic of Georgia? In the 1970s, Alexander Leaf, a prominent Harvard physician, wrote an article for *National Geographic* in which he described the extraordinary life spans of these mountain dwellers. There were healthy Georgians alive and kicking at 120, 130, and even 140 years of age. *Everyone,* from top scientists to everyday Joes and Janes, wanted to know their secret to longevity. Was it life at high altitude, diet, or a particular form of exercise? Was it, perhaps, the mountain soil, enriched by melting glaciers? On the basis of this last theory, millions of dollars' worth of supplements were sold here in the United States, with claims that minerals from glacial soils held the key to longevity.

There's one problem with this supplement and the "evidence" behind it: for all the scientific inquiry into the cause of the longevity in the Caucasus Mountains, no one—not even the esteemed Harvard doctor—had checked the facts. As it turned out, the people in these remote villages *weren't* living to 130 or even 110. These long-lived villagers were draft dodgers from World War I, when Russia was drafting all males 18 to 65. So these resourceful people added a few decades to their real age and claimed they were too old for military service. Their longevity wasn't caused by breathing thin air or eating goat's-milk yogurt, or growing crops in glacially enriched soil. It was "caused" by lying!

Yet you'll still hear certain supplement manufacturers boast that their products are backed by "evidence" from the Caucasus Mountains—or by similar (and similarly untrue) tales about the Hunzas in Pakistan or the village of Vilcambamba in Ecuador. If you don't know the facts, the stories about these long-lived villagers sound highly convincing, perhaps convincing enough to get you to buy a few bottles of pills. That's one reason I wrote this book: to give you the facts and help you draw smart, unbiased conclusions.

So how did I come up with the recommendations in this book? By doing what your doctor lacks the time to do: sifting through thousands of articles in top peer-reviewed medical journals. Below, I've listed the principles that guided me as I delved into each study. When you understand the philosophy behind my analysis, you'll be prepared if you ever come across an intriguing but unverified story like the one above, or if you need to make decisions about alternative treatments not specifically covered on these pages.

But if reading about scientific standards just isn't your cup of tea, that's fine. This chapter also contains my advice about buying supplements, talking to your doctor about alternative medicine, and under-

standing the most popular alternative therapies. Feel free to skip ahead
to these sections if you prefer.

TRY THIS WEBSITE

I've read thousands of medical studies so that you don't have to. If you're
interested in learning more about alternative medicine, however, one excellent and user-friendly resource is the website for the National Center
for Complementary and Alternative Medicine (www.nccam.nih.gov).

The Gold Standard

The gold standard for scientific testing is the double-blind, randomized,
placebo-controlled study (also known as an RCT, short for "randomized, controlled trial"). In an RCT, neither the subjects nor the doctor
know who is receiving the therapy being tested and who is receiving a
placebo (an inert look-alike). Subjects are carefully screened for the condition to be treated and then are randomly selected to receive either the
real therapy or the placebo. Without these safeguards in place, the
study's results could reflect conscious or unconscious bias by the investigators or the subjects.

I've relied on these well-controlled studies whenever possible. Unfortunately, this kind of rigorous testing is time-consuming, complicated, and
expensive. It also works better for studying pills and supplements than for
the long-term effects of behavioral choices, such as diet and exercise.
That's why I often look to good observational studies, which usually track
a group of people through several years or even decades, attempting to uncover any links between behavioral choices and specific health consequences. The best observational studies examine behaviors (eating several
servings of fruits and vegetables each day) or taking supplements, com-
paring them with health outcomes (heart disease or cancer).

A further challenge for RCTs is finding an adequate placebo for hands-on treatments such as acupuncture, massage, and chiropractic techniques. Sometimes you will have to make decisions about an alternative product or service in the absence of an RCT or a good observational study. I'll come back to this subject later.

The Best Journals

I give much more weight to studies that are published in one of the top-tier American journals, such as the *New England Journal of Medicine,* or in distinguished Western European journals, such as *The Lancet.* The editors of high-quality journals have done most of the legwork for us, checking the quality of the study and looking for conflicts of interest. Lesser journals, especially those that exist to serve a specialized branch of the alt-med industry, may have lower standards for publication. Some will print just about anything, including last week's grocery list.

Study Location

Many of the studies cited by health-store clerks and other alt-med enthusiasts have been performed in far-off countries. The United States and most other developed countries set their scientific standards high. Other countries don't always measure up. Some have neither a tradition of clinical trials nor an effective overseeing scientific body. In a few places, politicians are notorious for their willingness to arrange studies with outcomes guaranteed to please their sponsors—for a price. When I was traveling in China to study the traditional medicines there, health officials approached me with these offers on a frighteningly regular basis.

TOO GOOD TO BE TRUE?

The journal *Rheumatology* reviewed thirty-six published studies of acupuncture that were performed in China. Every single one was positive! Contrast this with the forty-seven American studies of acupuncture under review. Here, the results were positive about 53 percent of the time—a much more believable outcome.

Although I'm glad to see enthusiasm from Chinese scientists for their traditional medicine, I'd feel better about the quality of their evidence if at least *one* negative report for acupuncture came out of the People's Republic.

Wanted: Real Humans

I've witnessed this scenario too many times to count: a therapy, either conventional or alternative, is proven to fight off cancer cells, restore lost memory, or work some other wonder—but only in the artificial environment of a laboratory. When the same substance is tested on walking, talking humans, the treatment fails. Sometimes a nasty side effect rears its head. Next time you hear a claim that begins, "This herb has been proven to work in laboratory studies . . . ," ask yourself: Do I really want to ingest a substance based on how well it performed in a Petri dish—or in the body of a rat?

Size Matters

I'm always on the lookout for "proof" that comes from a suspiciously small group of subjects. How large does a study need to be? It depends on the effect you're trying to measure. Say, you're testing a potential treatment for a swiftly fatal disease. If you give this treatment to 10 people with the disease and they all live for another five years, congratulations! It's likely that you're on to something. But if you're looking for a more subtle effect, such as relief from arthritis pain, you'll need positive results from a much larger group of subjects before you can be sure the treatment works.

When Good Studies Aren't Available: Making Real-Life Decisions

Between those alternative therapies that have been proven by well-controlled studies to work and those that have been proven *not* to, there are many treatments whose effectiveness remains unknown. Some "remedies" are backed by little more than anecdotes of healing. Other claims are derived from a few poorly conducted or very small studies. No one has proven that they work, and no one has proven that they don't work, either.

Some medical experts believe in using only those products and services that have been proven by randomized, controlled trials. But given the limited state of funding for good research of alternative medicines, I find that reasoning overly restrictive. In fact, I use some unproven treatments for my own chronic ailments.

For example, in addition to some of the proven alternatives, I love therapies such as hydrotherapy and massage for my arthritis and back pain, even though they have never been tested in an RCT for either problem. Even in the absence of well-conducted studies, these therapies make good sense. I know that heat (in hydrotherapy) and tissue manipulation (in massage) can relax the hard knots of muscles that form around painful joints. I also advocate yoga and tai chi, whose gentle motions can help you move through your day with greater ease. These alternative therapies feel so wonderful and have so few side effects that I can't imagine even the coldest of rationalists would deny a pain sufferer their considerable comforts.

However, you will see that I strongly advise you to stay away from many other unproven treatments. What if, for example, the supplement that's been shown to work on guinea pigs turns out to be dangerous for long-term use by humans? Or if an herb that appeared to improve the memory of a few people in India interferes with your heart medication? When there are so many excellent alternatives out there, it just doesn't make sense to risk wasting your money—and your health—on those that are unproven, risky, and expensive. I've applied this practical logic to the treatments discussed in this book. Whether I recommend or reject a therapy, I explain the reasoning behind my conclusion.

BY ANY OTHER NAME . . .

Not everyone uses the term *alternative* to describe treatments that exist outside of med-school curricula. Many employ the word *complementary* to describe treatments that can be used alongside conventional medicine. The federal government's National Center for Complementary and Alternative Medicine uses both terms. Some practitioners object to these two labels, complaining that they don't give alternative medicine equal footing with prescription drugs and surgery. They prefer to speak of their therapies as *integrative medicine.* In this book, I've stuck with *alternative,* not out of a particular philosophical stance but because this is the term that most health-care consumers know and feel comfortable using. But I do believe that many of the alternative treatments in this book are complementary to traditional medicine and should be integrated into conventional medical care.

Supplements: Who's Looking Out for You?

Nearly all of alternative medicine exists in uncharted territory, but supplements present a special challenge for the consumer. The federal government does not classify supplements (including herbs and vitamins) as drugs. Instead, they are regulated the same way foods are regulated, which is to say that the Food and Drug Administration pretty much leaves them alone unless a substance is frankly dangerous. Supplement manufacturers aren't required to perform risk-benefit analyses or to undertake postmarket surveillance, as drug companies are. They don't even have to prove that the ingredients inside the bottle match the label on the outside.

So whom do you ask if you have questions? There is little guidance available that is both informed and unbiased. Few doctors and pharmacists are educated on the subject. By contrast, clerks at the health stores are more than willing to discuss the myriad products on their shelves. They have brochures and lots of anecdotes to share with you. But you may be uncomfortable—and rightly so—with taking health advice from someone without a medical background, or who may receive a commission based on how much you spend in the store.

Germany has a much more logical system. In 1979, the German Ministry of Health established Kommission E, a committee of twenty-four experts, to review botanical drugs and preparations from medicinal plants. Over the next fifteen years, Kommission E reviewed more than 300 commonly used botanicals for both safety and effectiveness. When it is relevant, I've drawn on Kommission E's work in this book—though many of its findings apply to proprietary supplements available only in Europe.

Where and How to Buy Supplements

Although there are no guarantees when it comes to supplements, a little consumer know-how will increase your chances of getting a product that is pure, accurately labeled, and safe. For the tips below I'm indebted to Gale Bensussen. Mr. Bensussen is president of Leiner Health Products, the largest supplement manufacturer in the country. Here is his advice:

LOOK FOR USP CERTIFICATION. In November 2001, the United States Pharmacopeia (USP), a nonprofit group, began its Dietary Supplement Verification Program (DSVP). Under this program, manufacturers of dietary supplements can submit their products for voluntary testing. If the product meets DSVP requirements for accuracy in labeling, purity, and good manufacturing practices, it is granted a USP certification mark. Look for it on the products you buy—but bear in mind that this mark does *not* indicate safety or efficacy of the supplement.

BUY FROM COMPANIES WITH THE MOST TO LOSE. Few health stores intend to mislead or defraud anyone. Because they are usually small businesses, however, they rarely have the infrastructure to properly assess the quality of their products. Internet sources can be even less reliable; it's all too easy for online peddlers of herbs to close up shop and vanish into the ether if their practices are called into question.

On the other hand, the larger drugstore and discount chains make easier targets if a product they sell turns out to be harmful or mislabeled. For this reason, they are often very careful. Many of these retailers are accustomed to working with supplement companies on safety and efficacy; they often have quality review boards that set standards for potency and hazard control, with a third-party laboratory to audit their products. Every year, they go to their own shelves and pick out products at random for a quality review.

There's one exception to this rule of thumb: If you are searching for a more esoteric product, such as huperzine A, or a newly popular supplement, you may have difficulty finding it in the drugstore or discount chains. In this instance, you're better off shopping at a health store. You may wish to try a franchise of a large health-store chain rather than going online or visiting an independent store for your purchases.

BIG CHAINS AND BRAND NAMES

Store brands are often a good bet for quality supplements. When big chains put their name or the store's private label on a product, the last thing they want is for that product to show up in the headlines of the *Wall Street Journal* or the *New York Times* because of contamination or mislabeling—so these supplements are usually put to a thorough test. (Remember that these tests are for purity and for accuracy of labeling, not for effectiveness.) Below are some of the biggest chains and their private-label brand names:

Chain	Brand Name
Costco	Kirkland Signature
Safeway	Select
Sam's Club	Member's Mark
Wal-Mart	Spring Valley

PERFORM YOUR OWN DISSOLUTION TEST. Your body can't absorb a pill that doesn't dissolve properly in your gastrointestinal tract. But many supplements don't disintegrate, meaning that they do not break up into smaller pieces. To test a pill, simulate stomach conditions by making a solution of equal parts vinegar and water. Leave the pill in the solution overnight. If it hasn't disintegrated by morning, toss the whole bottle. Better yet, return it to the store and demand a refund.

Even when you follow these suggestions for buying supplements, the big questions remain unanswered: Does this product really work? What are the side effects? Could it interact with any of your prescription medications? Similar questions haunt alternative services such as acupuncture, massage, and homeopathy. Some (though not all) of these fields have training and licensing requirements for their practitioners, but you may still lack the unbiased information you need. Is there good proof that this service will improve your problem? Is the service safe? Is it worth the money you're asked to pay?

This book attempts to answer these questions whenever possible. When sufficient information isn't available, I give you guidelines for making good judgment calls.

A Short Course in Alternative Therapies

Below are some of the most popular therapeutic systems covered by the umbrella term *alternative medicine*. Although I will occasionally introduce other treatments, this list describes those that come up most often in the pages ahead.

ACUPUNCTURE

Acupuncture is based on ancient Chinese theories about the way energy moves through the body. According to traditional Chinese medicine, this energy, known as chi, flows through invisible channels called meridians; certain points along these meridians help keep the energy moving properly. Disease occurs when energy is blocked at one of these points, or when it is moving too quickly or slowly. By inserting needles into the appropriate points, an acupuncturist can restore energy flow—and, theoretically, restore health.

That's the Eastern view of acupuncture, but many Western scientists have wondered if acupuncture might work in less mystical ways. Some have posited that acupuncture stimulates the body to produce higher levels of its natural painkilling chemicals. Others wonder if it affects levels of certain neurotransmitters.

One problem with acupuncture is that it's impossible to conduct a blind trial of its effectiveness: How do you come up with a placebo for needles, one that prevents both the subjects and the researchers from knowing which group is getting the real treatment? Some scientists have tried giving their study's control group something called "sham acupuncture," in which the needles are placed in spots *other* than those in which they are supposed to work for a particular ailment. But it turns out that even sham acupuncture has some effects! Nevertheless, this therapy has shown some interesting results in studies of certain disorders, especially arthritis.

When performed correctly, acupuncture is extremely safe. Just be absolutely sure that your practitioner is licensed to practice where you live and that he or she is certified by the National Certification Commission for Acupuncture and Oriental Medicine. It's even better if your acupuncturist holds a postgraduate degree in the field or is a licensed physician. *Always* be sure that your practitioner opens a fresh pack of disposable needles to use during your session. If you come across an acupuncturist whose office is dirty, or who uses old needles, run the other way.

AROMATHERAPY

Try sniffing a pencil eraser: the scent will take you straight back to first grade. Or breathe deeply as a peach cobbler bakes in the oven—you may feel as if you're standing in Grandma's kitchen. Aromas are definitely powerful stuff. But trips down memory lane aside, can aromas have a healing effect on your body? Specialty and health stores offer lavender to improve sleep, peppermint for sharper mental clarity, and ylang ylang to increase sexual desire.

If you enjoy these therapies and feel that they help you, that's good news. Aromatherapy is cheap, safe, and fun to use. There isn't much evidence that scents affect physical conditions, though, so use aromatherapy only as a pleasant adjunct to proven treatments, not as a substitute for them.

CHIROPRACTIC MANIPULATION

Chiropractors use highly physical techniques that move a joint past its range of motion—and out of its comfort zone—to its anatomical limit. That's why you hear a crack or pop when a chiropractor is working on you, and that's why you might feel some temporary pain as well.

There aren't many well-controlled studies of chiropractic treatment, and there's little convincing evidence that it can help back pain or other problems. But it's only fair to point out the challenges in creating RCTs of chiropractic treatment: as with acupuncture, it's difficult to create a placebo for this technique. A strong advantage of chiropractic therapy is that it involves a hands-on approach to healing. Some people find this a reassuring change of pace from the more clinical environment of a conventional doctor's office.

If you decide to try chiropractic treatment, ask your practitioner to use mobilization therapy, which is performed at a lower speed than high-velocity manipulation. The latter carries a very small risk of some very big side effects, including spinal compression and loss of bowel or bladder control. Never let anyone perform spinal manipulative therapy around your neck; there's a chance, albeit an extremely low one, that a stroke will result.

Your chiropractor should hold a doctor of chiropractic degree and be licensed to practice in your state. Beyond that, you'll want to be wary of any chiropractor who suggests very long courses of therapy, wants to sell you supplements, or recommends a series of expensive X-rays. These may not be necessary.

HERBS AND SUPPLEMENTS

Plants, not pharmaceuticals: that's the romantic promise behind herbs and other supplements. Manufacturers of supplements like to claim that their products are gentler, safer, more natural, and more effective than prescription drugs—and in some cases, they're right. To name a few instances: Saw palmetto can ease the symptoms of prostate enlargement with fewer side effects and less expense than conventional drugs. Calcium is one of the most effective PMS treatments around. Glucosamine and chondroitin are safer for arthritis relief than Celebrex—and they may go beyond pain control to actually halting the disease's progression.

As you might have suspected, however, there are plenty of other supplements that are toxic, risky, or simply useless. I'll talk about those in detail as well. As a general rule, remember that *natural* isn't synonymous with *safe*. Nature is a source of deadly poison as well as glowing health, so make sure that any product you take is backed by proof of safety— and that you get your doctor's approval before using it. Don't rely solely on the advice of health-store clerks or friends or yoga instructors or even herbalists.

A final note on herbs and supplements: many regions of the world have developed their own herbal traditions. Western herbal medicine, Ayurvedic medicine, and Chinese traditional medicine are the most popular in the United States today. How do they differ from one another? Western herbalism tends to prescribe herbs individually, matching an herb's effects with the patient's disorder. In their countries of origin, Ayurvedic and Chinese herbs are prescribed in complex mixtures that are prepared only after a long consultation with a doctor. I generally do not advise people to take Ayurvedic and Chinese herbal combinations that they find premixed and sitting on a shelf. Sometime these preparations contain herbs such as ephedra, which can be fatal. And we Westerners lack the expertise to properly analyze these combinations for interactions among the herbs. Please don't interpret this caution as a dismissal of Ayurvedic and Chinese traditional medicine. Both systems have been successful in their respective countries at maintaining health and well-being. My reservations are about their proper use and evaluation in the United States.

HOMEOPATHY

In the early 1800s, the German physician Samuel Hahnemann gave himself a small dose of cinchona bark, a substance used to make a cure for malaria. Hahnemann, who was healthy at the time, noted that this small sample of cinchona produced the symptoms of malaria in his body—but not the disease itself. From this observation, Hahnemann developed a system known as homeopathy, based on the principle of *like cures like.* Over a lifetime, he observed the symptoms that other substances produced in healthy people and used those substances to treat the same symptoms in the sick. Today's successful vaccines are based on a variation of this theme. So far, so good.

Hahnemann also claimed that smaller doses led to more effective treatment. He took this idea to the extreme, diluting his remedies to the extent that no trace of the active substance remained in the final product. Most homeopathic remedies you can buy in the health store today are totally inert. Yet homeopathy is included in the national health-care systems of Germany and the United Kingdom, and millions of people worldwide feel that homeopathy has helped them conquer chronic illness.

Some homeopathic practitioners claim that this therapy works by means of an energetic imprint left by the original substance; others simply say that they acknowledge a certain level of mystery. I, along with most other scientists, attribute homeopathy's popularity to a mind-body effect. And why not? There's nothing wrong with using a treatment that works via your mind, especially if that treatment is as gentle and devoid of side effects as homeopathy.

Although homeopathy is about as safe as it comes, it's not always cheap. The remedies themselves cost only a few dollars, but studies show that people who report the highest levels of relief are the ones who consult with a homeopathic practitioner. Perhaps that's because homeopaths create an individualized prescription for their patients—but more likely, this healing effect is generated by the long consultation session in which the homeopath spends nearly an hour discussing your symptoms and asking questions about your body, temperament, and life. Because a homeopathic consultation takes so much time, it also tends to cost real money. Be aware that most states do not have licensing standards for homeopaths, so you'll have to rely on word of mouth and your own good instincts.

HYDROTHERAPY

Here's a millennia-old therapy you can really sink into. The ancient Romans, who were well aware of the healing properties of natural hot springs, built whole villages around these important geological places. For many centuries, well-heeled Europeans have traveled to springs at places such as Baden-Baden, Vichy, and Marienbad to take the therapeutic waters. Today, millions of Americans avail themselves of the healing powers of warm water via their hot tubs, Jacuzzis, bathtubs, and showers.

No, there haven't been many clinical trials of hydrotherapy, but do you really need hard scientific evidence before enjoying a good soak? It stands to reason that plunging yourself into warm or hot water can relieve muscle spasms and stiffness, or wash away your stress after a tough day and help you sleep. (But stay away from very hot baths or saunas if a medical condition, such as cardiovascular disease or multiple sclerosis, makes overheating a danger for you.)

MASSAGE

Massage is the systematic manipulation of the body's muscles and soft tissues. This rather cold definition leaves out an important benefit of massage therapy: It feels great! Massage has not been put to rigorous testing for most disorders, but when your nerves are jangled or your muscles are painfully clenched, an experienced massage therapist can relax your mind and loosen your tight spots.

I prefer to hire a physical therapist to perform massage whenever possible. These experts have been trained to provide more than a relaxing experience; they know how to locate your trouble spots and when to avoid body areas that *shouldn't* be manipulated. Most states allow you to visit a physical therapist without a doctor's prescription, although there are advantages to checking in with your doctor first, as insurance companies will often pay for massage if it is part of a comprehensive treatment plan. When a physical therapist isn't easily available, look for a massage therapist who is licensed by your state. If your state doesn't require licensure, then the therapist should have passed the national exam for massage therapists, given by the National Certification Board for Therapeutic Massage and Bodywork.

MIND-BODY THERAPIES

Mind-body therapies may seem like a New Age trend, but most civilizations throughout history have relied on mental techniques to increase bodily health. Although each mind-body technique is different, they are often studied as a group. Below are some that come up in the chapters that follow:

BIOFEEDBACK: In this technique, your body's responses to stress are translated into visual or audio cues. By "seeing" your muscle tension as a series of waves on a screen or "hearing" beeps that indicate your body's temperature, you can learn to control these bodily responses—and possibly reduce pain, control stress, and improve sleep. Although biofeedback is painless, it does have a disadvantage over most other mind-body treatments: it requires an investment of time (usually several sessions with a specially trained physical therapist or psychologist) and possibly money, depending on whether your insurance carrier will reimburse you.

COGNITIVE-BEHAVIORAL THERAPY (CBT): You can't always control life's curve balls, but you *can* control your response to them. That's the guiding principle behind cognitive-behavioral therapy. CBT is a short-term, practical form of psychotherapy that helps you identify exaggerated or irrational thoughts and replace them with responses that are more realistic. So "I've been such a bad person that I deserve to suffer from back pain" might become "My pain has nothing to do with my past; I'm going to focus on living well today." Likewise, "I shouldn't have to deal with heart problems at my young age" is transformed into "Like it or not, I've been diagnosed with heart disease, but I can take several steps to improve my health and remain active." CBT is especially useful for anxiety and insomnia.

Theoretically, any psychotherapist should be able to help you use CBT, but it's best to find someone who is experienced using CBT for your specific health problem. Ask your doctor for a referral, or call the psychiatry or psychology department at a good university. Like biofeedback, CBT requires several sessions, but health-insurance plans will often cover the cost.

GUIDED IMAGERY: Guided imagery (sometimes known as visualization) uses the imagination to produce physical changes. Just by thinking of the aroma of tomatoes and garlic simmering in olive oil, for example, I can increase my saliva and stomach secretions. Proponents of guided imagery believe this therapy can lead to even more powerful effects. For example, women preparing for childbirth are often taught to imagine a "happy place," a relaxing mental scene that they can retreat to during labor pains. Cancer patients are sometimes told to visualize sharks or other predators who troll their bloodstream, gobbling up cancerous cells. This therapy can indeed help you find a drug-free way to alleviate anxiety, find a state of mental quiet, and perhaps allow you to distract yourself from pain. If you have a serious and progressive condition like cancer, it's fine to use guided imagery if it helps you feel empowered or relaxed, but never let it substitute for medical care.

MEDITATION AND THE RELAXATION RESPONSE: When Herbert Benson's book *The Relaxation Response* was published in 1975, its account of meditative activities and their effect on health propelled it onto best-seller lists across the country. Benson's technique, which he called "the relaxation response," does not require meditation as you and I might imagine it. You don't have to sit at the bare feet of a maharishi, for one. Nor does the technique need to be performed with crossed legs, over-whelmingly fragranced incense, and unwavering attention on a mono-syllabic "om."

Instead, this self-care technique provides a way to harness the mind's energy and direct it toward goals such as relaxing the body and decreasing your stress hormone levels. For more information, see the box below. You can also take courses that are offered in more traditional forms of meditation.

HOW TO ELICIT THE RELAXATION RESPONSE

In his book *The Relaxation Response,* Herbert Benson explains that the relaxation response requires two essential components: repetition of a word, phrase, image, or activity, and a passive disregard for any thoughts that interrupt this repetition. So you might sit in a comfortable position and do one of the following:

- Say a meaningful word, perhaps *peace* or *quiet,* aloud or silently.
- Say a prayer, if you're a person of faith, also aloud or silently.
- Think of a visual image, such as a candle lighting the darkness.

Then repeat this word, series of words, or image. If distracting thoughts come into your head (and you can be sure they will), resist the temptation to follow them. Don't punish yourself for having these

(continued)

wandering thoughts, either. Benson recommends that you say, "Oh, well," and calmly return to your word or phrase. Do this for 10 to 20 minutes. You'll know you've achieved the relaxation response when your mind is quiet and focused—instead of racing around from one worry to another.

Some people find it difficult to sit still like this. They may have better luck eliciting the relaxation response through physical activity. You can run, swim, knit, embroider, or do yoga while focusing on your breath or on the pattern of your movements. Just remember that if you find your mind wandering, you should refocus in a relaxed, nonjudgmental way.

TAI CHI

You've probably seen people practicing tai chi in a local park or even in a gym. This ancient Chinese exercise has recently become popular in the West, and for good reason: its gentle, steady movements encourage a meditative-like state that can transport you out of your day-to-day worries. Even better for the frail or elderly, tai chi improves balance— meaning that you are less likely to suffer a devastating fall. It also reduces the fear of falling, which can be even more disabling. Ask around to find a good teacher, or learn from a DVD or videotape.

YOGA

Yoga incorporates physical exercise, breathing and relaxation techniques, and meditation into a single pleasurable therapy. There are few good studies on yoga's reputed ability to cure disease, but try it anyway. You'll loosen up tense muscles, learn a variety of strategies for relaxation, and perhaps (depending on the type of class) even get your heart pumping. I recommend yoga most enthusiastically for arthritis, but it can be great for any medical condition with a stress-related component. And who doesn't find chronic health problems stressful?

You can learn yoga by watching a DVD or video, though I recommend taking a class at least once or twice to be sure you're using proper form. Inquire around town to find a good teacher. A great person to ask is your health-store clerk!

Working with Your Doctor

A few years ago, I took a trip to the Chinese province of Sichuan to study the traditional medicine practiced there. As I walked into a local hospital, I was nearly overwhelmed by the smells emanating from the first floor's large pharmacy. Instead of the rows of neatly labeled pills one might expect, the pharmacy overflowed with herbs, roots, stems, flowers, and even ground-up animal parts. Quite a change from the Lysol-scented corridors of Western hospitals.

I made my way into a room where a local practitioner was at work, administering one of these smelly concoctions to a patient and talking with him quietly. Although the room lacked the electronic monitors and other technical equipment that are de rigueur at home, I could sense a healing atmosphere in the room.

Then I spotted the IV drip.

"I don't understand," I said to the doctor. "Why is that here? Isn't traditional Chinese medicine based on herbal mixtures and acupuncture?"

"That's right; you *don't* understand," he replied. "Here in China we use the best of the East *and* the best of the West."

I share this humbling story as a reminder that *you* don't have to choose between conventional and alternative medicine, either. Like the people of Sichuan, you can take from the best of both worlds. A study by David Eisenberg and his colleagues at Harvard Medical School shows that most Americans already do. In a survey of 831 adults who used both conventional medicine and alternative services, more than 79 percent felt the combination was superior to either one by itself.

Count on your physician to diagnose problems, to assess underlying conditions that may require conventional treatment, to prescribe drugs and physical therapy—and to review *all* the alternative therapies you're using. For this purpose, you don't need your doctor to love alternative medicine; you just need someone who will check any supplements you're taking for potentially dangerous interactions and who will tell you when a therapy is inadvisable for your individual needs.

Set yourself up for a productive talk with your doctor by framing your questions so that they are as specific as possible. Questions such as "What do you think of alternative medicine?" invite a dismissal of the entire topic. Instead, try asking questions like these:

- I'd like to try Korean red ginseng instead of Viagra. Is it safe for me to take this herb?
- Is there any reason I shouldn't try massage therapy for my achy shoulder?
- I know you'd like me to reduce my risk of another heart attack by managing my stress. Can you refer me to a biofeedback specialist who can help me do this?

With these specific questions, you're much more likely to get a thoughtful, thorough response. Take this book to your appointment with your doctor. Point out the reference section in the back, which will help him or her locate the most relevant journal articles for the alternative therapy you'd like to try. (If a doctor is unwilling to entertain *any* discussion of alternative medicine, it's time for you to find another doctor.) After you've received an all-clear from your physician, you can turn to alternative providers like acupuncturists, homeopaths, massage therapists, and others for their specialized services, if necessary.

———

Now that you have some basic information about alternative medicine in hand, let's take a look at several chronic health concerens, reviewing the products and services you should avoid—and those that could significantly improve your life.

2

Joint Pain:
Improving Function,
Easing Discomfort

WHAT YOUR DOCTOR HASN'T TOLD YOU
AND THE HEALTH-STORE CLERK DOESN'T KNOW
ABOUT ALTERNATIVE MEDICINE FOR ARTHRITIS

What Your Doctor Hasn't Told You About Alternative Medicine for Arthritis	And What the Health-Store Clerk Doesn't Know
A combination of glucosamine and chondroitin sulfate can relieve arthritis pain and may arrest joint degeneration.	The dosages most likely to help you experience the benefits of these supplements
Acetaminophen (Tylenol) is not a great source of joint-pain relief.	Which therapy *does* reduce the pain of flare-ups and is available (free!) in your own home
Acupuncture can help reduce arthritis pain.	How often you need to receive treatments
The topical cream capsaicin can block pain signals by inhibiting Substance P.	There are products that can reduce capsaicin's unpleasant side effect.
	(continued)

What Your Doctor Hasn't Told You About Alternative Medicine for Arthritis	And What the Health-Store Clerk Doesn't Know
White willow bark has pain-relieving effects for arthritis sufferers.	This herb can be more irritating to your stomach than aspirin or ibuprofen.
Extracts from two common plants have been shown to provide significant arthritis pain relief with no known side effects.	Which other "joint health" supplements are a waste of money
You'll find much more information about these therapies—as well as many others—in the rest of this chapter.	

Like millions of other Americans, I suffer from osteoarthritis pain. Having begun my lifelong love affair with skiing in the era before safety bindings, I got a jump (so to speak) on arthritis in my teens by damaging several joints during less-than-graceful falls. Now, when I get out of the car after driving a long distance, I feel like the Tin Man from the Wizard of Oz—badly in need of an oil can to lubricate my aching joints and help me get moving again.

Most people use the term *arthritis* to designate a specific kind of joint pain known as osteoarthritis, and I'll do the same throughout this book. Arthritis is a common disorder—more than 20 million Americans have complaints related to this condition—and is caused by wear and tear to the cartilage within your joints. (Cartilage is a soft, semigelatinous material that covers the ends of bones and permits smooth, gliding interactions between them.) Over the course of a lifetime, normal activities such as walking place continuous, day-in, day-out strain on your joints, slowly damaging the cartilage and wearing it down so that the bony surfaces are exposed and rub against one another. The result: joint pain.

Oddly enough, the degree of joint degeneration doesn't always correspond to the level of pain a person experiences. For example, if you took X-rays of everyone over the age of 65, *nearly every single person* would show signs of osteoarthritic damage to their major joints. Yet—obviously—not everyone in this age group has joint pain. Some people have X-rays showing so much damage your hair would stand on end, but they report no pain or disability whatsoever. Other folks show few joint changes on their X-rays, but they have so much pain and stiffness that it's difficult to perform simple duties such as getting dressed or walking to the mailbox. I fall somewhere in the middle. My X-rays are really ugly, and I do have pain, but I can still play three sets of tennis or eighteen holes of golf.

Because I worry about the potentially damaging side effects of long-term use of pain medications like ibuprofen and acetaminophen, I try to minimize my reliance on them. I can't use Bextra or Vioxx, since the FDA took them off the market. Yet I continue to play several sports, not to mention hold down the simultaneous jobs of professor, clinician, author, husband, and father of four. Sometimes I hurt, but I've found methods—both conventional and alternative—to help me handle the pain.

As you probably know all too well, there is a bewildering array of products that claim to reduce arthritis pain or even reverse the condition. A short walk down the supplement aisle could leave your shopping cart piled high with products, from glucosamine to MSM to white willow bark. And what about all the flyers posted on the community bulletin board, the ones that advertise acupuncture or massage to soothe your hot, inflamed joints? You could spend the rest of your life—and your savings account—trying to find the best treatments! Not to mention that some of these so-called remedies could have serious health consequences. In this chapter, I'll help you sort out what works, what doesn't, and what just isn't worth your money.

ACHE ALL DAY, UP ALL NIGHT

If your arthritis pain keeps you up at night, you may find that the treatments suggested here relieve your discomfort so that you can rest. But you may also want to read chapter 4, "Satisfying Sleep," for insomnia-specific treatments that'll help you get the deep slumber you need.

Conventional Medicine: Surprising News

Doctors are taught to recommend acetaminophen (Tylenol) as the first line of treatment for arthritis pain. Up until very recently, it was believed that acetaminophen was as effective as many other pain relievers and had fewer side effects. However, a landmark trial conducted by Rush Medical College in Chicago and published in the *Archives of Internal Medicine* has shown what many arthritis sufferers already know: acetaminophen may be no better than a placebo at relieving the pain of arthritis. And at high doses, it can cause kidney disease.

Most people with arthritis turn to another category of medications for relief: nonsteroidal anti-inflammatory drugs (NSAIDs, pronounced *en*-saids). This category includes over-the-counter preparations such as aspirin, ibuprofen (Advil, Motrin), and naproxen (Aleve, Naprosyn), which do bring down pain levels but can also cause serious potential side effects. These side effects include peptic ulcer disease, gastrointestinal bleeding, and bleeding within the brain, which can lead to severe neurological problems and even death. Regular use of these drugs increases the risk of side effects, as does taking the drugs in excess of the recommended dose. Understandably, most people would prefer to find an alternative to leaning heavily on NSAIDs.

During the last decade, many arthritis sufferers have relied on COX- 2 inhibitors, which reduce pain and inflammation with less stomach irritation and blood thinning. Unfortunately, what has brought many sufferers into the health store is the bad news on Vioxx, Celebrex, and Bextra. Each of these brand names is a COX-2 inhibitor, and for several years all three were touted as nearly miraculous alternatives to aspirin and ibuprofen, because they relieve pain with fewer digestive side effects. But as so often happens, other—and uglier—effects began to appear after these drugs had been on the market for a few years. Now we know that people who take COX-2 inhibitors for more than eighteen continuous months are at a slightly higher risk for heart disease and stroke. And like other NSAIDs, long-term use can cause kidney failure.

There are some people who may nevertheless benefit from COX-2s. Folks with disabling arthritis pain (and no known risk factors for heart disease) may find that COX-2s are the only drugs that give them enough relief to get exercising again. In this case, the small risk of heart disease from NSAIDs is probably outweighed by the heart benefits of cardiovascular activity. But the FDA has pulled two of the leading COX-2 inhibitors (Vioxx and Bextra) off the market and placed a serious warning on Celebrex that might deter many physicians from prescribing it. As a result, it is hard to get a COX-2 drug nowadays.

Some other conventional treatments for arthritis pain are scary-sounding, but you should know that these techniques can change your life for the better. For example, injections of hyaluronic acid, a component of connective tissue, can replace a molecule found in joint fluid to help with shock absorption and lubrication. It's currently used mainly for knee joints, especially when NSAIDs aren't providing relief.

Corticosteroid injections can also work well to reduce pain and improve function. For many (though not all) sufferers with severe joint pain and swelling, corticosteroid injections into inflamed joints can provide relief for weeks or even months, but most people experience longer-term pain relief from injections of hyaluronic acid.

Surgical interventions are another possibility. Just be sure that you have examined all the other options. Once again, I'll use myself as a case in point. About twelve years ago, I had arthroscopic surgery on my left knee to remove debris from the affected joint. After the surgery and subsequent rehabilitation therapy, my joint pain diminished and its function improved. This left a lasting and important impression on me: I became a real fan—not of surgery, but of physical therapy. I realized that what had really helped me was not the painful insertion of a tube into my knee but the strengthening exercises I performed during rehabilitation to build up my lower extremities. Whereas my joint had once been suffering all the stress caused by walking and bouncing, my newly strengthened muscles were now able to absorb some of this burden, giving my knee additional support. The same principle applies to other joints as well.

I spoke with other doctors who agreed that weight training significantly reduces joint pain, and since then I've adhered religiously to my weight program. I've helped many people throw away their canes by encouraging them to buy weight machines or gym membership. (I'll come back to the subject of weight training soon.)

I was therefore intrigued by a study conducted by doctors at Baylor College of Medicine. In this study, 180 patients with osteoarthritis of the knee and pain that did not respond to medical treatments were randomly assigned to either receive arthroscopy or to have a simulated procedure. The placebo group with the simulated surgery went into the operating room, had their knees prepped for surgery, received mild anesthesia, breathed pure oxygen, spent the night in the hospital, and were treated as if they'd had a procedure performed. The shocking result: there was no significant difference in the knee pain between the two groups at any time after the surgery or the placebo procedure. So think twice, or at least get a second opinion, before you have arthroscopic surgery to relieve knee pain.

But don't swear off all joint surgery yet. There are good reasons to have joint surgery, such as the trimming of a badly torn meniscus, the spongelike disk in your knee joint between your thigh and calf bones that cushions the shocks on this joint. I had this surgery many years ago, and thanks to it I was able to resume tennis and skiing. There may also come a time when the joint surfaces of your knees or hips are so damaged that you can no longer walk without serious pain—and you'll feel more than ready to have these joints replaced. Technology has come up with some very effective artificial hip and knee joints that together with minimally invasive surgery have allowed people to quickly resume an active life. However, there are some complementary therapies that can prevent the need for surgeries in the first place.

You Can Prevent Arthritis—and Keep Current Joint Damage from Getting Worse

If you've just begun to notice achy joints, or if you're pain-free and hoping to stay that way, there's good news. You can postpone and perhaps even prevent osteoarthritis with some simple, proven measures. Most of you are unlikely to hear about these strategies in your doctor's office—but not because the evidence for them is poor. The evidence is actually quite sound and has been published in important medical journals. The reason you might not hear about them is that our health-care system doesn't permit doctors much time for talking to their patients about prevention.

The gurus hawking their alternative medicines on late-night television don't get such great marks on arthritis prevention, either. Many of them are too busy trying to wangle that last dollar out of your wallet to say, Hey, have you thought about getting some exercise or losing some weight?

The most obvious preventive technique is also the easiest: take commonsense measures to avoid accidents that cause joint injury. So buckle your seat belt, drive automobiles equipped with the latest safety features, such as side-impact air bags, and strap on your wrist and knee pads (or other protective gear) before playing rough-and-tumble sports.

Getting—and staying—strong is a less obvious but still vital way to ward off arthritis. Weight training strengthens the muscles around your joints, bolstering them against serious injury and subsequent damage. In one study at the Indiana University School of Medicine, just a small increase in the strength of the quadriceps muscle (that's the big muscle in each thigh) resulted in a 30 percent reduction of the risk of developing arthritis in the knee joint. Let's put this into perspective: if you go to the gym today and find that you're not so strong—maybe you can barely lift 5 pounds with your legs—all you'd need to do to reduce your risk of arthritis is to get strong enough to lift 15 pounds. (If you've never lifted weights before, that may sound like a lot, but most people discover that 15 pounds is a relatively easy burden when lifted with both legs. As a point of comparison, I regularly lift 60 pounds.) Even if you already suffer from joint pain, weight training can help you get around more freely. I lift weights three times a week for that very reason. You'll want to get approval from your doctor and then check in with a physical therapist or personal trainer to learn the best moves for your own painful joints. You may experience some muscle soreness around the joints at first, but within a few weeks of regular weight training (performed two or three times weekly), you'll notice that your arthritis pain is less bothersome. You can also perform aerobic exercises and stretches, which help prevent joint pain from starting—and from getting worse once it sets in. (Note that moderate exercise rarely causes joint problems, although extreme workouts—such as marathon training—can lead to injuries and pain.)

You may also need to lighten the load on your joints. If you're overweight, consider the burden you're asking your joints to bear: for each pound of extra weight, the strain across your knee joint increases by 2 to 3 pounds. Carrying 20 extra pounds around the middle means 40 to 60 additional pounds of stress on your poor, overworked knees. You don't need to diet yourself down to a stick to see results: Overweight women who lost just 11 pounds reduced their risk of developing arthritis with pain by half.

Adequate intake of both vitamin C and vitamin D can also protect you from arthritis. Although vitamin C pills are perennial best-sellers, there is little evidence that they provide the same protection against arthritis (as well as other conditions such as heart disease, cataracts, and cancer) as the natural compounds found in food. Just a glass of orange juice and a single serving of broccoli will provide the 250 milligrams of vitamin C you need daily to protect not only your joints but also your heart and eyes.

Vitamin D can be obtained by exposing your skin to sunlight, but if you live in cities (including New York, Philadelphia, Chicago, and Seattle) that are above 40 degrees latitude north or south, you do not get enough sunshine in the winter to make any vitamin D. Furthermore, many of us follow the good advice of our dermatologists and stay out of the sun or wear sunscreen, which interferes with the skin's ability to make vitamin D. To make things even more difficult, many Americans do not drink milk, the main food fortified with vitamin D. It is therefore not surprising that vitamin D deficiency is the most common vitamin

---

SEVEN EASY WAYS TO PREVENT ARTHRITIS (AND REDUCE YOUR PAIN)

1. Wear a helmet, knee pads, wrist guards, or other protective gear when playing sports.
2. Buckle up when in the car.
3. Avoid performing the same motion over and over as part of your daily routine.
4. Get 250 milligrams of vitamin C and and 1000 IU of vitamin D daily.
5. Start a weight-loss program (if you are overweight).
6. Pump some iron.
7. Get 30 minutes of moderate exercise at least five days a week, and stretch regularly.

deficiency in America. The best way to get the 1000 International Units (IU) of vitamin D a day you need may be through a supplement. The typical multivitamin contains only 400 IU.

It's unclear whether vitamins C and D can reverse existing arthritis or halt its progression. But since these vitamins make good health sense for your heart, bones, eyes, and other parts, why not incorporate them into your daily regimen?

The Discriminating Consumer's Guide to Arthritis Alternatives

Want to play golf again? Play the piano or type at the computer keyboard with less pain? Discover a backup therapy (or two) that will pull you through the rough days without extra drugs? Alternative medicines can help you accomplish these goals. I don't want to leave you with the impression that they will relieve all the aches and pains of arthritis, but neither will prescription or over-the-counter conventional medications. Used judiciously and intelligently, many of these alternatives can let you welcome former pleasures back into your life. Of course, many so-called arthritis treatments are all hype and little substance. I'll be more than happy to point these money-wasters out to you in the following pages.

HIGHLY RECOMMENDED ALTERNATIVE TREATMENTS FOR ARTHRITIS

Glucosamine and Chondroitin Sulfate

If you've got arthritis, you've probably heard of glucosamine and chondroitin sulfate. They have been used for decades in veterinary medicine to relieve joint pain and function, and since the 1980s European physicians have used glucosamine to treat human osteoarthritis. Both supplements stormed American shelves in 1997 with the publication of a book called *The Arthritis Cure,* which was emblazoned with the irresistible subtitle *The Medical Miracle That Can Halt, Reverse, and May Even Cure Osteoarthritis.* The book, which hailed both glucosamine and chondroitin as joint-healing wonder twins, became a certifiable sensation. In 1998, the year after it was published, more than 1 billion capsules containing glucosamine were sold in the United States. Alas, there's no proof that either glucosamine or chondroitin can *cure* arthritis, but there is increasing evidence that glucosamine and chondroitin sulfate can effectively relieve arthritis pain and stop the disease's progression.

In a controlled study published in the *Archives of Internal Medicine,* 200 patients with knee osteoarthritis were given either glucosamine or a placebo; all received X-rays every year for three years. When the study was complete, the X-rays from the patients who'd received a placebo showed a slow but steady narrowing of their joint spaces (caused by the loss of cartilage from bone surfaces). But those who took glucosamine showed *no* significant joint narrowing. It looks as if glucosamine can stop osteoarthritis in its tracks.

What about chondroitin sulfate? For many years, the media hype has belonged to glucosamine, and many people wondered if chondroitin was added to glucosamine to bring more money to the supplement manufacturers. But now we know that the case for it may be even stronger than for glucosamine, as a number of studies indicate that it reduces the pain and inflammation of osteoarthritis.

I take glucosamine and chondroitin sulfate every day and they've had a significant effect on the arthritis in my knee and shoulder. My knee and shoulder pain is gone and I can play my beloved tennis and golf and generally get around without too much difficulty.

DOSAGE: The recommended dose of glucosamine is 1500 milligrams daily. Since glucosamine is available in 500-, 750-, and 1000-milligram preparations, you can take the full dose at once or spread it throughout the day. Those with delicate stomachs should take glucosamine with meals. When taking glucosamine in pill form, I prefer the 750-milligram tablets that can be taken once in the morning and again at night. Many people, however, find the 750- and 1000-milligram pills difficult to swallow. Coated tablets can make the pills go down a little easier. Another alternative, albeit an expensive one, is a liquid formulation. But perhaps the best option of all is glucosamine in a powder. It's easy to take and is priced on a par with pills. In the mornings, I like to stir the powder into a smoothie made from skim milk, bananas, strawberries, and ice. If the powder makes your smoothie too sour, you can always toss in a teaspoon of sugar or sugar substitute to improve the flavor.

When buying glucosamine, you'll notice that it's available in several forms: glucosamine sulfate, glucosamine hydrochloride, N-acetyl, or chlorhydrate salt. I advise taking glucosamine sulfate, since most of the promising clinical studies have been conducted using it.

You'll need to be patient with glucosamine. It can take between four weeks and three months before its effects kick in. One review article published in the *Journal of Arthroplasty* suggests that relief continues for two months after stopping the product. You will probably need to take this supplement on a continual basis.

There is one important caveat when buying glucosamine: when scientists examined glucosamine levels in fourteen different commercial capsules and tablets, they found that the amount of glucosamine in the product varied from 41 to 108 percent of the amount stated on the label. To improve your chances of getting an honestly labeled product (and the best chances for relief), see the tips for buying supplements starting on page 8. Glucosomine is sometimes prepared from shellfish sources, so read the labels carefully if you have a shellfish allergy. Because glucosamine breaks down into glucose in your body, diabetics should speak to their physicians before taking glucosamine.

I also recommend taking 1200 milligrams of chondroitin sulfate daily. You can take all 1200 milligrams at once or divide that dose into two or three portions across the day. Again, the pills are so large that it's difficult to swallow comfortably; capsules or coated tablets can help the process, but powder or liquid formulations are other options. (Often, chondroitin is packaged with glucosamine. It makes no difference whether you take them together or separately, as long as you find a good product with the appropriate amount of both substances.)

As with glucosamine, you may need to take chondroitin one to three months before seeing positive effects. Both glucosamine and chondroitin can cause mild stomach irritation, so take the supplements with food if you have a sensitive digestive system.

Capsaicin

Capsaicin is the chemical responsible for the zing in hot chili peppers and paprika, and it can also produce good relief from arthritis pain. This natural compound, available at most pharmacies as well as health stores, is applied to the skin over the painful joint. It is believed to work by depleting one of the neurochemicals responsible for transmitting the pain sensation, appropriately named Substance P. Many people swear by the effects they get from capsaicin, but some swear *at* these effects—and I'll explain these different reactions.

It's hard to perform double-blind, placebo-controlled trials for capsaicin, because in some people the compound produces an easily identifiable stinging sensation when applied to the skin (yes, that's the reason for all that swearing). Nevertheless, several clinical trials have shown that capsaicin reduces arthritis pain. In one nationwide, multi-site study, 101 arthritis patients received either capsaicin cream or a placebo that looked similar but did not sting. They were all instructed to apply the cream four times a day. After four continuous weeks of treatment, the patients using the capsaicin cream reported pain reduction of anywhere between 33 and 57 percent, far beyond what the placebo patients reported. Imagine cutting your present pain by one-third or one-half. That can make the difference between playing eighteen holes of golf or watching golf on television.

Capsaicin's only real side effect is that stinging sensation, but some people don't experience the stinging at all. Others don't mind it and actually find it kind of pleasant; they compare it to Ben-Gay. But about a third who use a smaller dose (cream with 0.025 percent capsaicin) and more than half who use a higher dose (cream with 0.075 percent) report a really uncomfortable burning feeling. Again, some prefer this sensation over arthritis pain and some get used to it—but there are those who would rather go back to their Advil, thank you very much.

If you've tried capsaicin before and stopped because of the burning, here's some good news. We've known of compounds that can relieve the unpleasant sensation, but we have long wondered: if the burning stops, does the pain relief stop as well? The study I mentioned above appears to have answered that question. The study's researchers, wondering if the skin-tingling sensation itself played an important role in pain relief, took a closer look at the group who received capsaicin. They compared those who felt stinging with capsaicin use with those who reported no stinging. There was very little difference in their reported levels of pain relief, meaning that the burning sensation isn't a necessary part of capsaicin's pain-relieving effects.

This is good news, because it means you can take advantage of the compound glyceryl-trinitrate (GTN), which, when applied to the skin, helps relieve the discomfort capsaicin can cause. GTN is available over the counter and has pain-relieving and anti-inflammatory effects of its own when applied to the skin. In fact, the combination of capsaicin and GTN appears to provide more pain relief than the capsaicin by itself. Go easy on your use of GTN, as it can cause headaches. Another way to reduce capsaicin-related burning is to add lidocaine, a local anesthetic, to capsaicin. You'll need a prescription for lidocaine. If you want to try capsaicin, keep in mind that it has a cumulative effect, meaning that you need to apply it consistently—four times a day—for its pain-inhibiting work to kick in. That can be a serious commitment for some people. Unless money is no object, you may prefer to use capsaicin only on smaller joints, as it can be expensive to use enough capsaicin to cover the larger ones. Don't expect capsaicin to start blocking arthritis pain on the first application, either. Give this treatment several days before deciding whether it works for you.

DOSAGE: Start by applying a cream (one of the most popular brand-name capsaicin creams is called Zostrix) containing 0.025 percent capsaicin four times a day for four weeks. If you don't experience relief, try a cream that contains 0.075 percent four times a day. No matter which formula you use, wear gloves when you apply capsaicin and take care to keep it away from your eyes and other mucous membranes.

Acupuncture

Thanks to several interesting studies, most conventional doctors will prick up their ears if you mention acupuncture, even if they don't much care for alternatives in general. That's because they're at least vaguely aware that acupuncture has a fascinating history and tradition, and an impressively wide range of possible biological effects. One of the most popular—and scientifically supported—reasons for using acupuncture is arthritis pain. It's even received a stamp of approval from the U.S. government for use in conjunction with conventional therapies.

The National Institutes of Health have found the evidence for acupuncture as an arthritis therapy so compelling that in 1998, they released a consensus statement acknowledging that acupuncture releases the body's natural pain-relieving substances, called opioid peptides. These chemicals have potent effects similar to narcotic drugs such as codeine and morphine but without the same side effects of sedation, constipation, and dry mouth.

Since the government consensus, a number of small but high-quality studies have shown that patients felt significant pain relief when they received acupuncture in addition to conventional therapies for their arthritis-related knee pain. In these studies, patients received acupuncture twice a week for three to eight weeks—so if you want to try this therapy, plan on going two times every week for several weeks before you decide whether it works for you. You may also wish to try electroacupuncture (also known as Western acupuncture), in which gentle electrical stimulation is incorporated into the treatment.

If you try acupuncture and it helps relieve your pain, how long do you need to keep making trips to your friendly neighborhood acupuncturist? That's unclear for now. Although most studies showed that pain relief dropped off one month after the end of treatment, one study suggested that the pain-inhibiting effects of acupuncture could last for three months or even longer. Keep in mind that these studies showed no consistent evidence that acupuncture improved the *function* of arthritic knees. You may experience pain relief but still not feel like springing up the staircase two steps at a time.

Acupuncture's great advantage is its lack of side effects. Of course, you must be sure that the needles do not bring any viral or bacterial diseases into your body. But that's easily accomplished by visiting a reputable, licensed practitioner and making sure you see him or her open a fresh package of needles before treating you.

RECOMMENDED ALTERNATIVE TREATMENTS FOR ARTHRITIS

Avocado/Soybean Unsaponifiables (ASU)

True to my skeptical but always-curious nature, I was both surprised and excited when I found that avocado/soybean unsaponifiables (ASU) are more than just another unpronounceable arthritis gimmick. ASU is made up of a mixture of avocado and soybean oils—one part avocado, two parts soybean. This mixture is treated to remove some of the oils, which are used for making soap, and what's left is called unsaponifiables.

In a nicely conducted double-blind French study, researchers took 164 patients with painful osteoarthritis of the knee and split them into two groups. One received 300 milligrams of ASU every day for six months, and the other got an identical-looking placebo. The group receiving ASU reported a significant drop in pain and less need for other medications when compared with the placebo group. Although it took two months for the ASU to start relieving the pain, the relief lasted two months after the patients stopped taking the product. And there were no side effects.

Another high-quality trial of ASU, this time in Belgium, showed that people taking ASU reduced their need for NSAIDs (medications such as naproxen and ibuprofen). This study also established that a higher dose of ASU isn't necessarily better: 300 milligrams per day worked just as well as 600.

If you're wondering how this unusual combination of substances relieves arthritis pain, you're not alone. One exciting finding from Australia is that sheep that receive ASU are less likely to develop osteoarthritis than those that don't. This has led researchers to wonder if ASU protects joints from the effects of wear and tear. Some have speculated that ASU's active ingredient or ingredients are related to vitamin E and may act as antioxidants. Whatever the reason, ASU appears to work in these preliminary studies.

DOSAGE: 300 milligrams of ASU daily.

Transcutaneous Electrical Nerve Stimulation (TENS)

Most physical therapists are well equipped to outfit their clients with transcutaneous electrical nerve stimulation (TENS) units, so TENS is not, strictly speaking, an alternative therapy. I'm including TENS here nevertheless because so many physicians just don't think about TENS when they're prescribing treatment for arthritis. If you're interested in this promising therapy, you may need to inquire about it specifically.

TENS is a portable, wearable unit that conducts a mild electric current through the skin. A physical therapist usually works with his or her client to find a frequency and intensity of stimulation that inhibits pain without being annoying in itself. The client can then take the unit home and clip it to clothing, turning it on as needed. (The pain relief usually occurs only when the unit is in use.)

No one is exactly sure how TENS works, but there is some evidence suggesting that it releases opioids, the natural pain-relieving substances produced by the body. Others believe that TENS works because the sensation of electrical stimulation travels to the spinal cord more quickly than the sensation of pain, thereby "beating out" the pain for the nervous system's attention. TENS has been shown to work on back pain, shoulder pain, and knee pain, as well as labor pains, which should tell you something about its ability to handle heavy-duty discomfort! TENS is safe for most people, although it can interfere with pacemakers and other implanted electric devices.

Hydrotherapy

Whenever my arthritis reaches a high point, I stoke up the Jacuzzi and spend 30 minutes relieving my painful joints and muscles in one of the most pleasurable therapies around. Hydrotherapy is perfectly natural and feels terrific. A hot tub or Jacuzzi is particularly effective if you can maneuver the bubble-generating nozzle toward the affected joint or muscle. No, the pain relief doesn't always last very long, but hydrotherapy can often pull you through a bad day without your having to pop an extra pill. Hydrotherapy has no significant side effects, unless you have a medical condition, such as heart disease, that prohibits extended soaking in hot water. If you've never used a hot tub or Jacuzzi before, try it out for a just a few minutes at first, gradually extending your soak as you determine your comfort level.

Massage Therapy

Like a self-reproducing alien in a horror movie, pain spawns more pain. When you have joint inflammation, the pain can make your muscles grow tight and tense in response. Often they will clench into a spasm. You may have lived with this feeling for so long you don't even realize that your muscles aren't in their natural, relaxed state. And now you're stuck in the pain cycle, suffering from both joint *and* muscular pain—and possibly some insomnia thrown in, just to make life a little more challenging. This is a good time for therapeutic massage, which can break this cycle, reduce your pain, and help your muscles and mind relax. I've benefited from this treatment myself: when my arthritic hip flares up, I visit an expert massage therapist for prompt relief.

When you're shopping around for the right massage therapist, look for someone who is experienced with clients who suffer from osteoarthritis pain. The best possible choice is someone trained by a physical therapy program at a good university. If you're at one of those day

MORE MASSAGE FOR YOUR MONEY

Alternative medicine isn't really an alternative if you can't afford it. Here are a few tips for reducing the cost of massage:

- Avoid day spas and head for a private therapist instead. (Why pay extra for a fluffy bathrobe and an expensively manicured receptionist? Besides, day spas often save money by hiring therapists with less experience than private practitioners.)
- Ask if your health club has a massage therapist on staff; your membership fees may subsidize part of the treatment cost.
- If you live in a big city, consider traveling to the suburbs, where the rents are lower and so are the prices.
- Check your health-insurance policy. It may cover massage therapy if you use it for an approved condition. You may need your doctor's referral.

spas that offers a menu of massage choices—Swedish, Rolfing, myofascial release, shiatsu—don't feel flummoxed. There is no good information about exactly which kind of massage is best for arthritis, so choose a treatment that sounds good to you. If you've never had a massage before, you can just explain what your needs are. Don't let yourself get pressured into any extra-expensive treatments (you don't really need the package that features stones flown in from a sacred site in Bali, sprayed with incense, and lovingly warmed over an open flame), and again, request an experienced therapist. And if the massage causes pain to your arthritic joints, have the therapist stop immediately.

Yoga and Tai Chi

Some arthritis therapies, such as acupuncture, have been shown to reduce pain but not function or mobility—meaning that you might feel better if you use them but you won't necessarily be able to weed your garden or play Red Rover with the kids. That's why I'm delighted yoga and tai chi have become so popular. They not only reduce pain, they can get you moving again.

These light forms of exercise take pressure off your joints by building up the muscles that surround them. They also gently stretch out muscles and tendons that have constricted with pain and disuse, thereby increasing your range of motion. Both yoga and tai chi are deeply relaxing—some people feel that they are forms of moving meditation—and maybe that has some effect on pain and mobility, too.

I've talked to people who've been frightened off yoga by those photos—we've all seen them—of ancient yogis doing headstands and back bends. But rest assured that most beginners' yoga and tai chi classes are very simple and are designed for people who aren't human Slinkys. If you've got serious joint degeneration in your spine or neck, you may need to take a special rehabilitative class. Plenty of yoga studios, health clubs, and hospitals offer such instruction. And of course you should talk to your doctor first.

ACCEPTABLE ALTERNATIVE THERAPIES FOR ARTHRITIS

Ginger

You probably know ginger from stir-fries, sushi bars, and holiday treats, but this spice has also been used in India and China to treat musculoskeletal conditions for more than 2,500 years. How does it stand up to modern-day scrutiny?

There have been a couple of good studies on ginger. In the first, which was conducted at ten sites across the United States, 247 patients with osteoarthritis pain of the knee took either ginger or a placebo for six weeks. At the end of the trial, the patients who received the ginger reported significantly less pain while standing and walking, and less stiffness. They also noted some relatively mild gastrointestinal side effects, including a bad taste in the mouth, burping, upset stomach, and heartburn.

Enter the second study, performed in Denmark, in which ginger was compared with both ibuprofen and a placebo. This was a crossover study, meaning that patients took each of these three "treatments" at different times. This time, ginger produced pain relief that was only marginally better than the placebo and definitely far less effective than ibuprofen.

So what do I make of this information? Like garlic, ginger is a wonderful addition to many meals and may help soothe an upset stomach. I suggest using as much ginger as you like to improve the flavor of your food, but for arthritis pain I recommend using other remedies with better proof—at least until further studies on ginger are completed.

DOSAGE: Although I don't yet recommend ginger for pain relief, I understand that an informed consumer may wish to try a ginger product anyway. Since it's been taken for millennia with few reported ill effects, ginger is considered fairly safe. The usual dosage is 1 to 4 grams a day, spread out over two to four doses. It's best to use ginger from the Alpina or Zingiber plant genera, because these have been tested most often—but it can be difficult to track the source of herbal preparations, as I've noted before.

White Willow Bark (Salix alba, Salix purpurea, Salix fragilis, Salix daphnoides)

In the pantheon of herbs, white willow bark is often granted the status of a demigod. The Roman physician Galen used it in the second century B.C., and it's been a staple of traditional Chinese medicine for millennia. In the nineteenth century, white willow bark was such a widely used herb that European chemists decided to tinker with it a little and isolated its active ingredient, salicylic acid. Eventually the Germany company Bayer synthesized a derivative of salicylic acid, and now we all reach for aspirin instead of the trunk of the nearest white willow tree whenever we feel a headache coming on.

Actually, some people still do rely on white willow bark to reduce pain and inflammation (but they don't tear off strips of the nearest willow tree, they buy the product in packaged form). You may have heard claims that this herb isn't as harsh as aspirin or other NSAIDs. But this is one of those times when natural isn't necessarily better. The acid present in white willow bark is actually quite rough on the stomach, because of its high concentrations of tannins, astringent substances that can irritate the digestive system. In fact, the Bayer people developed aspirin because there was a need for something gentler than this herb. If you find that white willow doesn't bother you as much as aspirin does, it's probably because you're getting a relatively small dose, with an equally small effect on your pain.

DOSAGE: If you'd like to try white willow bark anyway, you can take the amount recommended on commercial preparations—but you should know that dosages for white willow have not been scientifically determined. Avoid this herb if you have bad reactions to aspirin or other NSAIDs, are sensitive to salicylates, or suffer from kidney problems, tinnitus (ringing in the ears), peptic ulcer disease, or any other conditions that prevent you from taking aspirin or NSAIDs.

Magnets

Aristotle recommended magnets for their healing properties. Cleopatra is said to have worn one encircling her forehead—or, depending on which history book you read, to have slept on one to preserve her youthful charms. Today, many sports stars will tell you that their joints—and playing ability—have been saved thanks to magnetic shoe inserts or other products. You may hear the claim that magnets stimulate nerve endings or help blood vessels carry more oxygen.

But there is little good research supporting magnet use for arthritis pain. The few studies that have been performed looked at very small groups of people, and the results have not been duplicated. If you'd really like to try magnets, however, you can rest assured that they are probably quite harmless. Just don't use them if you have a pacemaker or an implanted defibrillator, or if you're near someone who does, because the magnetic field could interfere with the operation of these devices. And whatever kind of magnet product you buy, don't invest a lot of money. Just go down to your drugstore or health shop and pick up something nice and cheap. Make sure that their strength is between 250 and 500 gauss (which is about fifteen to twenty times stronger than the kind of magnets that your mother used to hold your good report cards to the fridge). But your dollars and efforts would be better spent on therapies with better evidence.

DO NOT USE THESE ALTERNATIVE TREATMENTS FOR ARTHRITIS

Devil's Claw (Harpagophytum procumbens)

Many natural-healing guides and herbal "experts" promote devil's claw as a pain reliever and anti-inflammatory agent. But based on the evidence, I'm less than enthusiastic about this herb.

Several European studies have specifically examined the effects of devil's claw on osteoarthritis pain. Some of these studies looked at the effects of devil's claw versus that of a placebo, and others used NSAIDs as a point of comparison. The results showed some, but not much, pain relief—and that relief occurred only when people took the herb at high doses (and the study's authors were vague about how high these doses actually were). The response of some salespeople to these results is "Great! I'll start recommending high doses of devil's claw right away!" My response? Not so fast. For one, the pain relief showed in these studies was so minimal as to be statistically insignificant. Perhaps more important, I'm just not comfortable recommending that people take high doses of an herb we don't know much about. When there are so many really effective alternatives out there, why take the risk for such small results?

Articulin

Articulin is a popular Ayurvedic herbo-mineral complex that includes zinc and some exotic-sounding herbs: *Boswellia serrata* oleo-gum resin, *Withania somnifera* root, and *Curcuma longa* rhizome. Although articulin is touted as a wonder drug by some, I'd like to see better evidence and more information about possible side effects.

Here's what we know: In a study conducted in India, 42 patients were given either articulin or an identical-looking placebo. They received their treatment for three months, and then the groups were switched. According to researchers, patients reported reduced pain and less disability while taking articulin.

This is an intriguing finding, but I'd feel much better about it if these results had been repeated in the United States or Western Europe, where scientific controls are generally much tighter and more reliable. I'm watching this one closely—but you couldn't pay me to pop these pills before I know more about them.

MSM (Methylsulfonylmethane)

When the book *The Arthritis Cure* hit the stands touting glucosamine and chondroitin, other books soon followed with their own claims about so-called miracle drugs for arthritis. (I discuss glucosamine and chondroitin earlier in this chapter.) One of the most popular of these compounds is MSM, promoted in a best seller titled—you guessed it—*The Miracle of MSM*. This book proposes that MSM is "the first safe, natural, side-effect-free remedy for many types of pain and inflammatory conditions."

Since you've chosen to pick up *my* book, you're probably somewhat skeptical of breathless sales pitches such as the one above. When it comes to MSM, that skepticism is particularly well advised. There are simply no good scientific trials of MSM that either support or refute the extravagant claims made for this compound. You may have friends who will testify to the drug's healing properties, but I don't recommend using MSM until more is known about it.

Reumalex

When you're strolling down the "joint health" aisle at the health store, you're likely to find an herbal mixture called Reumalex. This product contains white willow bark, which contains salicin. It also includes poplar bark, which produces chemicals similar to willow bark—guaiacum resin, black cohosh, and sarsparilla, all of which are traditional Native American treatments for rheumatic conditions. If you ask a salesperson's advice, he or she may well recommend Reumalex; you may even have friends who've used it.

But I cannot advise you to take this product. When scientists in the U.K. performed a randomized study of 82 people with chronic arthritis pain, subjects who were given Reumalex did not report a significant decrease in pain when compared with those who received an identical-looking placebo. Save your money for those products and services that actually work.

Stinging Nettle Leaf (Urticae dioica)

Stinging nettle consists of leaves, either fresh or dried, of the urtica plant in its flowering season. These leaves have sharp spines that contain histamine, acteylcholine, serotonin, and formic acid, which irritate the skin when they are applied directly (hence the name). Like so many of the herbs described in this book, stinging nettle has a long tradition of medicinal use; in this case, both Native Americans and medieval Europeans employed it to reduce joint pain and improve other conditions. Present-day proponents of the herb say that the active ingredients listed above can safely relieve arthritis. Are they right?

To date, there's been only one reasonably well-conducted study of stinging nettle, and it was a pretty small study at that. At the University of Plymouth in the U.K., 27 patients with osteoarthritis were treated either with stinging nettle leaf or with an identical-looking plant called white dead nettle, which does not sting. The placebo group did not report much of a change after one week of use, while the patients using stinging nettle reported a decline in both pain and disability.

But I wouldn't put stinging nettle on my arthritis shopping list yet. The problem with these promising results is that the placebo, which is necessary for a really excellent study, wasn't such a good choice. It lacked the easily identifiable skin sensation that stinging nettle produces, so it was probably easy for the placebo group members to figure out that they didn't have the real thing. And unlike the researchers who performed the study on capsaicin (described earlier in this chapter), the researchers failed to measure whether the stinging feeling is necessary for any pain relief that stinging nettle might produce. This study is a good start and gives us further reason to study stinging nettle more closely. Until the evidence is better, however, stick with products that are known to do some good.

SAMe (S-adenosyl-L-methionine)

SAMe can be found in every cell of your body. It's a critical component of a number of biochemical reactions and is particularly important in the formation of certain neurochemicals. There is interesting speculation that certain disorders, such as Parkinson's disease and depression, are caused in part by a deficiency of SAMe in certain cells and that taking supplemental SAMe could help. In fact, Europeans have been taking synthetic versions of SAMe as a treatment for depression and arthritis for years. In Italy, it's even sold by prescription, under the name Samyr. Here it's sold as a dietary supplement, and a month's supply will set you back anywhere from $20 to $50.

In the mid-1980s, several clinical trials in the United States suggested that SAMe was as effective as NSAIDs (medications like aspirin and ibuprofen) in the treatment of arthritis. Based on this initial evidence—as well as on claims that it could improve depression, fibromyalgia, migraines, and liver problems—SAMe has become one of the top-selling dietary supplements in the country.

More recent studies of SAMe for arthritis pain have been disappointing, however. In these studies, SAMe has performed only slightly better than a placebo. Although it has fewer side effects than NSAIDs do, it can cause unpleasant digestive problems such as diarrhea. It also holds potential dangers for anyone with bipolar disorder, as it may exacerbate agitation and manic reactions in this population.

LABELS NEVER LIE . . . OR DO THEY?

The company ConsumerLab.com, which conducts independent tests of health products, tested thirteen brands of SAMe available in the United States. In six of those brands, the amount of SAMe in the pills was *less than half* the amount indicated on the label.

The lesson? Always remember that the supplement industry is relatively unregulated. Makers of your prescription drugs, beef products, and children's toys all must meet strict government standards or face the consequences, but supplement manufacturers have few restraints. For my advice about buying the best supplements, see chapter 1, "Shopping Smart for Alternative Medicine."

Not only are the test results conflicting; there is also much confusion surrounding the appropriate dose for SAMe. Some studies suggest 400 milligrams per day; others have concluded that you'd need 1600 milligrams each day to receive whatever benefits SAMe might have. The jury is still out on SAMe.

The Complete Prescription for Pain-Free Joints

MAINTENANCE
Glucosamine: 1500 milligrams daily
Chondroitin sulfate: 1200 milligrams daily
Yoga, tai chi, or stretching exercises: daily
Weight training: 2 or 3 times a week
Cardiovascular exercise: 30 minutes daily (5 days a week minimum)

TO CONTROL FLARE-UPS
Capsaicin: 0.025 percent capsaicin cream, four times daily for four
    weeks; increase to 0.075 percent capsaicin cream if needed
Acupuncture: twice weekly or as needed
Avocado-soybean unsaponifiables (ASU): 300 milligrams per day
    as needed
Ibuprofen or other NSAIDs: as needed
Massage therapy: as needed
Hydrotherapy (hot bath, hot tub, Jacuzzi, or hot shower):
    as needed
Transcutaneous electrical nerve stimulation (TENS):
    as needed

3

Back on Track: Relief for Back and Neck Pain

WHAT YOUR DOCTOR HASN'T TOLD YOU AND THE HEALTH-STORE CLERK DOESN'T KNOW ABOUT ALTERNATIVE MEDICINE FOR BACK AND NECK PAIN

What Your Doctor Hasn't Told You About Alternative Medicine for Back and Neck Pain	And What the Health-Store Clerk Doesn't Know
The best treatment for acute low-back pain is neither medication nor surgery.	Most acute low-back pain will disappear with almost *any* treatment.
Massage can relieve the muscle spasms that accompany back and neck pain.	One popular form of massage therapy can have life-threatening side effects for neck pain sufferers.
White willow bark may reduce or even eliminate some cases of back pain.	Its side effects can be rougher than those of conventional pain medications.
A treatment called percutaneous electrical nerve stimulation (PENS) may reduce back pain.	PENS appears to have its best effect when used with another therapy.
	(continued)

What Your Doctor Hasn't Told You About Alternative Medicine for Back and Neck Pain	And What the Health-Store Clerk Doesn't Know
Commercial heat wraps can cut down on back pain.	So can similar at-home treatments you can prepare for free.
You'll find much more information about these therapies—as well as many others—in the rest of this chapter.	

I worked my way through med school as a medical technician, a job that included drawing blood for clinical analyses. One busy day, when I was leaning over to draw yet another blood sample, I tried to straighten up . . . but couldn't. My back muscles were in spasm and I was stuck in a position that made me look like Quasimodo. I spent the next month on my back and strung up to a medieval-looking traction apparatus, with my feet attached by pulleys to weights in an attempt to straighten out my muscles and other tissues. Since then, research has shown that neither bed rest nor traction works for back pain. That month of my life was not only uncomfortable. It was wasted.

Luckily, Western medicine no longer treats back spasms with weeks-long bed rest and torture devices. Not so luckily, there are only a few conventional treatments that deliver consistent help without serious side effects. Most sufferers find that drugs like acetaminophen (Tylenol) aren't up to the task of relieving their pain, whereas stronger treatments like opiate medications leave them woozy or uncomfortable. Other treatments, such as surgery, have obvious risks with surprisingly few clear benefits. This situation dogs countless Americans for whom back and neck pain is a frequent companion. Five million of us are currently disabled by low-back pain alone.

As if back and neck pain weren't paralyzing enough in themselves, the number of alternative therapies that claim to heal these conditions could stop the most discriminating consumer in his or her tracks. In the following pages, I'll help you sort through the products and procedures available. I'm confident that you'll discover strong alternatives to strong medications—and surgery—for your pain.

Causes of Back and Neck Pain

It often happens like this: you twist or bend in a slightly odd way, or you pick up something heavy without bending your knees. Then you feel a telltale twinge along your spine or neck, followed by excruciating pain.

This scenario describes acute pain, which can last for days or weeks. Most people familiar with acute spinal pain just sigh and take the treatment that's worked best for them before, and then let someone else do the heavy lifting for a while as their pain recedes. And in fact, that's a pretty good plan of attack. About 80 percent of the time, acute back pain goes away by itself. (There are also some specific strategies for easing an episode of acute pain. I'll talk about these soon.) But if your pain persists for three months or longer, it's considered chronic. Chronic pain is more difficult to treat, and you'll have to become a savvy shopper of conventional and alternative remedies for your condition.

Science hasn't told us much about what goes wrong inside the back and neck during an episode of pain, whether acute or chronic. Sometimes—though not very often—the pain is a symptom of another problem. If you experience ongoing or recurrent pain, you'll need a doctor to rule out an underlying cause.

But don't be surprised if your doctor can't find a reason for your pain. Back and neck pain remain frustratingly mysterious. However, we now have some useful information about what *doesn't* cause the pain. Degenerated and herniated discs, once thought to be a major cause of pain along the spine, exist in many of us, but they don't necessarily lead to pain or disability. One study looked at people over the age of 60 who *didn't* have back or neck pain, and 64 percent of them showed some kind of disc degeneration on MRI scans. Even among younger people, asymptomatic disc degeneration is common: about 20 percent of folks under 40 who don't have spinal problems have discs whose inner core is bulging outward.

Although it's good news that degenerated or herniated discs don't always lead to a sentence of lifetime disability, it's unnerving when no one can figure out why you hurt so much. Luckily, it's not always necessary to know *why* a problem occurs in order to make it feel better.

My own life is a great case in point. I've suffered from back pain for years. Every weekday, I get up and drive my kids to their different schools, each in a different town. Then I drive to work in South Central Los Angeles, drive back home to Hollywood, take the kids downtown for music lessons, and drive to play dates all over the metropolitan area. Sometimes I'm in the car as much as three or four hours a day. The result is one sore back. I use a seat cushion and have a car with good shock absorbers, but I still need hydrotherapy (also known as my Jacuzzi) to keep my back relaxed. Since no two people experience pain in the same way, you'll probably need a different set of therapies to help you stay active. Read on to learn about several you can choose from.

WHEN BACK AND NECK PAIN SIGNAL AN EMERGENCY

Most cases of back and neck pain do not point to an underlying disorder, although the pain itself is undoubtedly unpleasant. But in a few instances, back and neck pain are signs of an emergency. If you experience any of the following, seek treatment from a physician immediately:

1. *Back pain accompanied by muscle weakness or numbness in the legs or feet.* These symptoms could indicate damage to the spinal nerves. You'll need to see a doctor right away to determine the site of nerve compression. From there, active intervention to relieve pressure on

(continued)

the nerves might be warranted, although in some cases your doctor may instead decide to monitor your neurological complaints closely.

2. *Back pain accompanied by pain or numbness in the genital or rectal area and/or urinary or fecal incontinence.* These serious symptoms can indicate cauda equina syndrome, in which the nerve roots at the lower end of the spinal cord are compressed. To avoid permanent paralysis and incontinence, a doctor must relieve the pressure on the nerves that are being compressed.

3. *Neck pain with numbness and weakness of the arms, hands, or fingers.* These symptoms can indicate compression of nerves in the neck. Again, you may need immediate surgery to avoid paralysis.

4. *Back pain that is not relieved or is made worse by lying down.* This may indicate a mass or tumor near the spinal cord.

5. *New back pain in people with cancer or osteoporosis.* The pain could reflect a progression of these diseases.

6. *Pain that spreads to both arms or both legs.* Symmetrical pain in the limbs could indicate one or more serious conditions.

Conventional Medicine for Back and Neck Pain: Minimize Your Risk of Side Effects

In the last few decades, conventional medicine's arsenal against back pain has been nearly depleted. Studies show that once-common treatments such as a corsets, back braces, and traction (my personal nemesis) are ineffective. Most doctors no longer use them, and you should stay away from those who do. Until a few years ago, bed rest was also standard advice for an episode of back pain, but now we know staying in bed is just about the *worst* thing you can do. If you experience acute back pain, you probably won't feel like exercising—if your back locks up, as mine did in med school, you may not be able to—but you should move as much as you reasonably can. After a few days, it's best to resume most of your normal activities, aside from work that puts a serious strain on your back.

Among the remaining conventional options, pharmaceuticals stand nearly alone as proven treatments for back or neck pain. That's one reason why 80 percent of initial doctor visits for back pain conclude with the doctor handing over a prescription. Unfortunately, drugs often bring problems of their own. Aspirin and nonsteroidal anti-inflammatory drugs (NSAIDS, which include Advil, Aleve, and Motrin) are popular for garden-variety back pain, but they can also cause gastrointestinal bleeding. This fearsome side effect kills thousands of Americans every year. Other risks include bleeding inside the brain, peptic ulcer disease, or aggravation of preexisting asthma. Your chances of incurring these side effects are much higher if you take more than the recommended amount of the product—which is worrisome, given that most sufferers will admit that they need a higher daily dose to keep their pain under control.

I know many people who request muscle relaxants from their doctors when acute pain twists them into agony. Stay away from these drugs, however, because there's little evidence that they are better than a placebo, and they can cause drowsiness and dizziness.

As I mentioned in the previous chapter, COX-2 inhibitors—once a drug of choice for pain relief—have been found to increase heart disease risk, especially when taken for more than eighteen months in a row. Two of these popular medications (Bextra and Vioxx) have been pulled off the market, and you may find that your physician is reluctant to prescribe Celebrex, the remaining available brand.

If you've been thinking that you want a gentler approach to pain relief, you're thinking smart. On these pages, I'll show you treatments that are kinder to your entire body.

Steroid epidural injections are often recommended for treatment of moderate to severe back pain, but they have no benefit over placebo injections for chronic back pain. The one exception may be for low-back pain accompanied by sciatica, which is a burning pain that runs down the lower back and into the thigh and leg.

Will I need surgery? That question nags at the minds of back- and neck-pain sufferers, appearing with the first knifelike slice of acute pain and growing louder as chronic pain takes its toll on daily life. What you and your doctor may not realize is that spinal fusion—a popular form of back surgery in which the spinal vertebrae are welded together—is not much more effective than exercise in treating back pain. Obviously, surgery also comes with potential complications, such as infection, bleeding, and the risks related to anesthesia. Before you agree to surgery, have a long talk with your doctor. Some procedures have a good track record with particular kinds of pain; others amount to nothing more than a desperate last resort. In the latter instance, less drastic measures usually work just as well or better.

The Discriminating Consumer's Guide to Alternative Medicine for Back and Neck Pain

Ready to snap into your skis this winter? Or to pick up your adorably wriggly grandchildren? I hope so, because alternative medicine holds the closest thing we have to a cure for back and neck pain.

But the alt-med field is also chock-full of treatments that will waste your time and money. Here's a fact to keep in mind as you shop around: except for one or two marvelous exceptions—which I hope you'll try— most back-pain alternatives haven't been proven to work any better than a placebo. Does this mean you need to avoid these alternatives? Not necessarily. The placebo response for back and neck pain is very high, meaning that if you believe a treatment is going to work, it probably will. We know from clinical trials of acupuncture and massage that patient expectations can determine the effectiveness of each procedure: patients who expected acupuncture to be highly effective indeed reported less pain after acupuncture, whereas patients who thought massage would bring them relief responded better to a rubdown.

I know people—both doctors and patients—who take this news to mean that massage and acupuncture are scams. Those people are missing an essential point: a treatment that safely reduces back or neck pain is a successful treatment, no matter what the reason. If chronic-pain sufferers feel better, they *are* better. (Of course, this isn't true for other disorders, such as cancer. A massage during cancer might help a person feel better, but that wouldn't mean the tumor had disappeared.) That's why I encourage you to follow your impulses when it comes to alternative medicine for your back or neck pain. If you are attracted toward a safe but unproven therapy such as homeopathy or massage, try it! You are making a smart decision to engage your mind's healing power to its fullest capacity. Of course, I don't recommend you throw reason out the window. Use your head and the information in this chapter to determine which treatments are safe and most appropriate for your condition. And don't go bankrupt pursuing an expensive but unproven treatment.

A final word of caution: remember to make your physician a part of your pain-relief team. Although we can't always pinpoint the source of

THE PUBLIC'S PREFERENCE

According to a national survey conducted in 2003, nearly 65 percent of sufferers rated massage as "very helpful" for their back and neck pain. Chiropractic manipulation and relaxation also scored high with sufferers. None of these therapies has been proven to consistently reduce back and neck pain in clinical trials, and evidence strongly suggests that chiropractic treatment *isn't* effective. Yet people ranked these therapies far higher than the services of doctors, who received a "very helpful" rating from only 27 percent of patients. Not only does this survey indicate that the human mind can wipe away pain, it also shows that we physicians just aren't doing enough for the millions of pain patients who come to us for relief.

your pain, it's important that we check things out, just in case the causes can be identified. The medical journal *Spine* reported the case of a 68-year-old woman who suffered back pain that radiated to her backside and thigh. She received acupuncture treatment for a year before the unrelieved pain drove her, finally, to see a conventional physician. Her doctor ordered an MRI, which revealed the cause of her pain: a mass near her spine that pressed on her nerves. She had surgery—and when the mass was gone, so was her pain.

HIGHLY RECOMMENDED ALTERNATIVE TREATMENTS FOR BACK AND NECK PAIN

Exercise

To be blunt, there aren't many alternative therapies for back and neck pain that have actually been proven to help you. But now I can show you hard proof that your pain can be greatly reduced—and even eliminated—with a home-based and free treatment.

For chronic back and neck pain, a specialized program of exercise is the very best medicine. Though exercise may not seem like an alternative medicine, it qualifies here because many physicians fail to recommend it to their patients with back pain, despite the evidence that it helps. These doctors are not necessarily uninformed, but they have often become discouraged over the years as their patients have made beelines away from their exercise regimens and toward their comfy couches.

I often suggest that pain sufferers try therapies that most appeal to them, provided those therapies are known to be safe. But not everyone finds the thought of exercise appealing—especially pain patients who are worried that exercise will make them feel worse or cause deeper damage.

If this describes your attitude, you'll have to pull up your socks and go *against* your instincts. A number of different exercise programs are great for back pain; they all include strengthening techniques for your abdominal, back, neck, and shoulder muscles. Although exercise programs sometimes cause additional soreness at first, they won't damage your back or neck if you perform them correctly. Instead, you will find yourself stronger and more limber than you've felt in years. Here are just some of the exciting studies proving the link between exercise and relief from back and neck pain:

- In 2001, the Philadelphia Panel (a group consisting of experts in medicine, physical therapy, exercise, rehabilitation, and family practice) concluded that the *only* treatment that worked for either back or neck pain was therapeutic exercise. The panel's definition of "therapeutic exercise" included stretching, strengthening, and mobility exercises.

- When neck-pain patients spent a year adhering to a program designed to strengthen the muscles in their necks, 73 percent reported total or considerable relief. This same study showed that aerobic training also had a good effect: nearly 60 percent of sufferers of this group found that their pain was gone, or nearly gone, after a year of workouts. By contrast, only 21 percent of patients in a control group experienced comparable relief. One unexpected finding from this study was that strength training increased range of motion and flexibility to a greater degree than aerobic training.

- If X-rays showing disk degeneration have left you fearful of exercise, here's some comforting science: thirty-five patients with low-back pain and herniated disks, degenerative back disease, and other back complaints were randomly placed in either an aerobic exercise group (which involved walking or cycling at a low to moderate intensity for 45 minutes, four days a week) or a control group that did nothing. After ten weeks, the exercising group reported significantly less anger, depression, and tension—and not one person suffered from new or in-

creased back pain while working out. But the most promising results occurred when the researchers checked in with the exercise
group two and half years later. Those who were still exercising
used fewer pain medications and visited the physical therapist
less frequently. They also lost less work time.

PAINLESS EXERCISE

If the thought of simply walking down the stairs makes you wince in
pain, you'll need to match your exercise to your body's needs. Here are
some gentler workouts that won't pound your sore muscles and aching
joints:

- *Brisk walking.* If walking on dry land is too painful, try using
  a warm-water walking tank to take the stress off your joints.
  These tanks are available in many physical therapists' offices.
  Ask your doctor to write you a prescription.
- *Swimming.*
- *Water aerobics.*
- *Cycling.* If back pain makes a regular bike too uncomfortable,
  try riding a recumbent bike instead.
- *Cross-country skiing* or *stationary ski machines.* These activities
  are aerobically challenging but aren't high-impact (unless, of
  course, you fall off your skis).
- *Elliptical trainers.* Another low-impact, whole-body workout
  available at nearly every gym. Just be sure not to slouch; keep
  your head up and your spine straight.

Sticking to an exercise program is challenging for many people, especially for those who wake up every morning in pain. If your doctor hasn't
written you a referral to a physical therapist who will get you started on
an individualized exercise program, ask him or her to do so now. Your

physician will probably be impressed with your interest in exercise, and the physical therapist can provide you with guidance, safety tips, and motivation. Here are some other tips to keep in mind:

- Don't overdo. Start off with a walk around the block or a slow ride on the exercise bike. Soon your body will acclimatize to the activity, and you can increase the duration and intensity of your workouts.
- Ice down the painful area before and after exercise. Fill a small paper cup with water and stick it in the freezer. When it's frozen, peel off the lip of the cup and rub the ice on the area that hurts. Or use an ice pack.
- Consider trying percutaneous electrical nerve stimulation (PENS, described later in this chapter), which may allow you to exercise with less pain.
- Enjoy the results! As your mood levels soar and pain levels plummet, you'll find yourself craving a good healthy sweat.

I recommend a combination of cardiovascular exercise, stretching, and strength training to reduce your pain. You should get about 30 minutes of cardiovascular exercise most days of the week. Don't worry about trying to keep up with the twentysomethings who spend hours sweating on the StairMaster; just find an activity you like and push yourself just enough that you start breathing deeply. If you're gasping for air or can't carry on a conversation as you exercise, you're working too hard.

Most people with chronic back and neck pain suffer from limited flexibility in the affected area. Whether this tightness is a cause or a result of pain is one of those chicken-and-egg questions. The important thing now is to perform stretching exercises that will increase your mobility and loosen up those pain-causing muscles.

Strength training is often neglected by fitness enthusiasts, but it appears to be the most important feature of a pain-control workout. Strengthening your abdominal muscles, for example, will take the burden off your aching back and protect you from further injury. And recall that study of neck pain, in which strength training produced total (or almost total) relief in 73 percent of the patients.

A good weight-training program won't include the kind of grunt-and-lift maneuvers you see at the Olympics. You don't need to look like Arnold Schwarzenegger. The goal is improved muscle tone, not muscle mass. If you have never been a fitness enthusiast, I strongly recommend spending a few sessions with a personal trainer or physical therapist *before* you pick up those weights.

RECOMMENDED ALTERNATIVE TREATMENTS FOR BACK AND NECK PAIN

Heat Wraps

You've probably seen advertisements for commercial wraps that adhere to your lower back or your neck and then produce a sensation of heat. One product was tested in a study of more than 300 patients with acute low-back pain. The patients were given one of the following: acetaminophen, a placebo, a ThermaCare Heat Wrap, or an unheated wrap. Then they were asked to rate their pain. The patients who used the heat wrap had more pain relief and were more likely to return to normal activity than the others in the study. (Ibuprofen came in second, followed by acetaminophen and then the placebo.)

This study has all the hallmarks of excellence: the patients were divided into groups randomly; there was a placebo control; and the study was conducted in several places, which lowers the possibility of bias. However, I should point out that this study was sponsored by Procter & Gamble, the manufacturers of this product, whose scientists also organized the research.

Certainly there's no harm in trying a commercial heat wrap. Swaddling your sore muscles in a toasty swath of fabric is undeniably comforting, and it makes sense that heat can coax some of the tension out of tight muscles. But you can achieve a similar effect with an old-fashioned home remedy: just fill an old, clean sock with rice and zap it in the microwave for 30 seconds. Be careful not to overheat the rice. You can then wrap the warm sock around your neck and shoulders, or place it against your lower back and relax in your favorite chair. If you want to wear a heat wrap as you perform your daily activities, though, or if you'd like to wear the wrap overnight, a commercially prepared product that clings to your body and stays hot (the ThermaCare wraps remain hot for eight hours) might be a better match for you.

Hydrotherapy

Perhaps the most ancient therapy for back and neck pain is balneotherapy—which is an impressive-sounding way to say "baths." Galen, the second-century Roman physician, recommended baths to his patients, and healing spas all over the world have flourished ever since. Although many sufferers will testify to the healing powers of baths, there's been surprisingly little research on their actual effect on pain.

Personally, I'm convinced of the restorative powers of a hot soak. It stands to reason that the warmth can relax muscles that have seized up in response to pain. A bath or shower also lets you take a break from the demands of the day—and that effect may be the most powerful of all. During an acute episode of neck pain, you might stand under a hot stream of water in the shower (don't scald yourself); if you're mobile enough, a trip to the tub or Jacuzzi could ease you through an acute bout of back pain. And any day that you feel tension creeping into your back or neck, consider yourself entitled to some hydrotherapy. You might just head off a more serious bout with pain.

Hydrotherapy is usually very safe, but there are a few people who need to avoid immersion in hot water, including folks with heart conditions. If you're new to hydrotherapy, don't jump straight into a very hot bath. Instead, start off with warm water and gradually turn up the heat until you find a comfortable temperature.

Massage

For back and neck pain, massage makes sense. No matter which tissues—joints, muscles, tendons, ligaments, nerves—are giving you grief, massage can loosen up the muscles that have undoubtedly grown tight in response to the pain. It's also a divinely relaxing therapy that— at least for me—can melt away a week's worth of overbooked schedules, long commutes, and even parent-teacher conferences. By reducing tension, you also reduce the chances that stress will deposit itself directly into your back or neck. Which is why it's so frustrating that no one has conducted a rigorous study of massage and its effects on back and neck pain. Although I can't provide you with strong evidence for massage, I nevertheless recommend you try it at least once, for the reasons given above. I usually ask for a standard therapeutic massage, ideally by someone with training in physical therapy, and skip the fancy treatments like Rolfing (which involves an often painful manipulation of connective tissue) or shiatsu. If you want to try something more exotic, that's fine, so long as you avoid shiatsu massages that focus on your neck. The journal *Neurology* reported two cases of patients who suffered life-threatening injuries to the blood vessels in their necks after receiving shiatsu massages.

Percutaneous Electrical Nerve Stimulation (PENS)

You may have heard of transcutaneous electrical stimulation (TENS), a form of physical therapy in which electrical simulation is applied to the skin in the hopes of relieving pain. Although I'm dubious about the positive effects of TENS for back pain, a new twist on this older therapy may hold more hope. This variation on TENS is called PENS— percutaneous electrical nerve stimulation. PENS also features low-intensity electrical stimulation, but in this case the stimulators penetrate the skin. As with acupuncture, there may be some discomfort, but it is minimal.

There have been several studies of PENS with positive results, although most trials are somewhat tainted by inadequate placebos. But in one excellent study of 34 patients with chronic low-back pain, one group received real PENS while the other got a sham form of PENS. Both groups also underwent a physical therapy program that featured exercises known to reduce low-back pain. After three months of treatment, the sham PENS group showed no improvement in their pain, while the patients receiving real PENS reported that their pain was cut nearly in half. Measures of performance (including the time required to rise out of a chair and the ability to lift objects) and depression both improved significantly with PENS, but not with the sham PENS. The authors of this study have suggested that PENS stimulates the release of endorphins near the spine, providing enough pain relief to permit effective physical therapy and exercise. Whether PENS is useful for neck pain remains unclear.

This therapy requires a certain tolerance for the time-consuming practice of finding just the right location for the stimulators and the frequency that produces the most relief with the least annoyance. You may have to visit your physical therapist several times before you hit on the right combination. But if PENS allows you to perform the exercises that will almost definitely help you feel better, it's worth the time investment. If you have an implanted pacemaker or defibrillator, you'll have to choose a different therapy.

ACCEPTABLE ALTERNATIVE TREATMENTS FOR
BACK AND NECK PAIN

Acupuncture
Although acupuncture isn't the most popular alternative treatment for back and neck pain (chiropractic manipulation holds that distinction), nearly everyone knows a sufferer who claims life would be unbearable without regular acupuncture tune-ups. In 1998, the National

Institutes of Health confirmed that acupuncture stimulates the release of opioid peptides, which are natural painkillers manufactured by the body. Acupuncture might relieve pain by stimulating the release of endorphins, the body's natural painkillers. Others believe that acupuncture prevents certain kinds of sensations from traveling up the spinal cord and into the brain, where noxious sensations are processed into the feeling of pain.

To everyone who finds relief from back and neck pain with a skilled acupuncturist and a pack of clean needles, I say: More power to you. But despite the tantalizing theories and the good news about acupuncture's effect on pain in general from the National Institutes of Health, the evidence for acupuncture's effects on low-back pain specifically is inconclusive. (The evidence for its use on arthritis is more compelling and is described in the previous chapter.)

There have been dozens of acupuncture trials for back pain. No matter what you might hear from acupuncture enthusiasts, however, you'd do well to ignore most of those studies, as they were sloppily conducted and used few controls. One scholarly review looked at the few studies that met basic scientific standards. Of these, four studies concluded that acupuncture worked—and two concluded that it didn't. Which is another of way of saying that acupuncture for back pain might work, or might not. Results for acupuncture on neck pain are similarly inconclusive.

For now, I'll speculate that the most genuinely therapeutic effect of acupuncture for back and neck pain may be the hands-on, caring quality of the treatment and the relaxing time spent on the acupuncture table. If you feel a strong connection to the philosophy behind acupuncture, it might be worth your while. At the very least, your belief and interest will increase your chances of triggering the placebo effect. And if you feel better, who cares whether needles or your mind is the cause?

If you are interested in acupuncture for back- and neck-pain relief, make sure you give the treatments plenty of chance to work. This means going twice a week for several weeks. As always when undergoing acupuncture, make sure the practitioner is licensed, keeps a clean office, and opens a fresh pack of needles in front of you before treatment. *Never* risk being stuck with a dirty needle.

You'd also do well to avoid a trendy variation on traditional acupuncture called local acupuncture. Although most acupuncture is fairly or even completely painless, in this therapy the acupuncturist intentionally places needles in the sites where your back or neck muscles are most sore. As you can imagine, this hurts like the dickens, and there's some posttreatment pain as well. And preliminary evidence indicates that it's less effective than regular acupuncture. I'd stay away from it.

Chiropractic Manipulation (for Back Pain)

Americans have a love affair with chiropractors. We are more likely to see a chiropractor than any other alternative-care provider. When it comes to low-back pain, we're more likely to see a chiropractor than a *doctor.*

Despite its popularity, chiropractic does not appear to be a useful therapy for back and neck pain. More than ten randomized and controlled studies of chiropractic manipulation on back pain have been published. Again and again, reviewers have concluded that chiropractic manipulation appears to be slightly more effective than no treatment at all, but when spinal manipulation is compared with other back and neck therapies, this therapy isn't all it's cracked up to be.

Any discussion of chiropractic reminds me of a classic episode of *The Simpsons,* in which Homer Simpson sits in an examining room listening to his long-winded chiropractor. Homer, still waiting for his manipulation, finally yells, "Less yakkin', more crackin'!" It's a great television moment, but I'd guess that most chiropractic patients enjoy their visits with a chiropractor who takes the time to talk and to listen. This unhurried, caring approach probably accounts for much of chiropractic's appeal.

If you suffer from back pain and like the idea of chiropractic, it's all right to try. Beware that chiropractors are notorious for prescribing long and expensive courses of therapy. ("You'll need to see me twice a week for the rest of your life" is a common joke among veterans of chiropractic treatment.) Go only for as long as you need to. If you get relief, that's terrific. Now use your newfound mobility to undertake an exercise program, or you'll land back in the chiropractor's office sooner than you'd like.

Manipulation of the back can cause temporary and mild pain—so if you are really hurting and unwilling to risk further discomfort, chiropractic may not be for you. There is also a much, much lower risk (ranging from one in one million to one in one hundred million) of compression of the spine and loss of bowel and bladder control. If you're going to try chiropractic treatment, ask your practitioner to use mobilization (performed at a low velocity) rather than manipulation (done at a high velocity). And never let a chiropractor touch your neck. [If you suffer from neck pain, see "Chiropractic Manipulation (for Neck Pain)" on page 76.]

If this information has made you nervous about chiropractic manipulation, but you still like the idea of hands-on healing, you may appreciate massage, physical therapy, or osteopathic treatment instead. These are discussed elsewhere in this chapter.

Osteopathy

Like chiropractors, osteopaths use spinal manipulation therapy. Unlike chiropractors, osteopaths are fully licensed physicians who can diagnose conditions and look for underlying problems. Is it worth making a special trip to an osteopath to treat your back or neck pain?

In a randomized, controlled study published in the *New England Journal of Medicine,* 178 patients with low-back pain were divided roughly into two groups. The first group received the usual conventional therapies—an assortment of aspirin, acetaminophen, NSAIDs, opioids, physical therapy, and so on. The second group was given osteopathic treatment. After twelve weeks of treatment, both groups reported the same substantial amount of pain reduction. The osteopathic treatment was less expensive and less likely to produce side effects. I'd like to see more studies of osteopathy before drawing final conclusions; until then, I rank it on the same level as chiropractic treatment. Osteopathy may be useful for back pain, but as with chiropractic, it's inadvisable to let anyone use forceful actions around your neck.

Look for an experienced osteopath—preferably one associated with a medical center—and one who enjoys a sterling reputation.

White Willow Bark (Salix alba, Salix purpurea, Salix fragilis, Salix daphnoides)

White willow bark is often recommended by alt-med types as an alternative to pain medications. Indeed there is some good evidence that it helps relieve back pain (the evidence for white willow bark's effect on arthritis, discussed in the previous chapter, isn't as strong). In one study published in the *American Journal of Medicine,* 210 patients with low-back pain were randomly assigned to receive one of three treatments: willow bark containing 240 milligrams of salicin (willow bark's active ingredient), willow bark containing 120 milligrams of salicin, or a placebo. After four weeks, 39 percent of the high-dose group was free of pain! In the lower-dose group, 29 percent reported cessation of their pain symptoms. Only 6 percent in the placebo group reported similar relief.

Before you try white willow, there are a few things you need to know. Although the chief appeal of alternative medicine is its claim to gentleness, white willow can be a bit tough on your gastrointestinal system. Aspirin was actually derived from white willow—and then buffered with other chemicals to ease the undesirable side effects of this herb, which include digestive irritation and gastrointestinal bleeding. And there's no evidence that white willow is *more* effective than aspirin or other NSAIDs, which also cause GI side effects. If you have any difficulty with NSAIDs, suffer from kidney problems, tinnitus (ringing in the ears), or peptic ulcer disease, or are sensitive to salicylates, don't take white willow bark.

DOSAGE: If you do wish to take white willow, you can try pills that yield 60 to 120 milligram of salicin a day divided in two or three doses. Start at the low end and slowly build up if necessary.

Transcutaneous Electrical Nerve Stimulation (TENS)

Transcutaneous electrical nerve stimulation (TENS) was developed about thirty years ago in response to a theory about the origins of pain perception. In this theory, known as the gate-control theory, pain perception can be altered or even prevented if other sensations such as touch or pressure can get in the way of pain, blocking it from moving toward the brain. By applying light electrical stimulation to the skin, TENS supposedly provides one of those alternate sensations and prevents its users from feeling quite so much pain.

Three decades later, both the theory and the therapy remain fascinating (though not adequately proven). And TENS does appear to work well for arthritis pain. But does it help sufferers of back and neck pain? For reasons that are unclear, TENS does not appear to help pain in these regions. An excellent review of five high-quality trials of TENS for chronic low-back pain showed no significant benefit over sham forms of TENS (which are usually much like TENS without the electrical current).

TENS is safe, however, as long as you don't mind the possibility of a rash at the site of the electrical stimulation pack that sits next to your skin. People with implanted pacemakers or defibrillators should not use TENS at all. If you're bent on trying TENS, plan on plenty of visits to the physical therapist, who will have to use trial and error to determine the site and frequency that seem to work best for you. (That's one reason TENS is rarely used for acute pain: by the time the equipment is set up and working at an optimum capacity, the pain has subsided on its own.)

You'll have the most luck if the stimulator is placed close to the site of your pain.

If you find TENS intriguing, consider a closely related therapy called percutaneous electrical stimulation (PENS), which is backed by stronger evidence for back pain. PENS is described earlier in this chapter.

Homeopathy

If your health store carries homeopathic remedies, you may have noticed that there are several items purported to relieve back pain. Before trying them, you should know that there are no rigorous studies to back up the use of homeopathy for back or neck pain, and that most scientists, including me, feel that homeopathy has little basis in science. That's because the ingredients are so diluted as to be nonexistent; the remedies appear to be little more than placebos.

They are also inexpensive and free of side effects, however, so there isn't a strong downside to experimenting with homeopathy if this therapy appeals to you. You can visit your favorite supplier of health goods, choose one of the remedies listed here, and take it as directed on the label.

If you find homeopathy attractive and want to maximize your chances of relief, you might have more luck visiting a homeopath for a one-on-one consultation. Homeopathy seems to have a better track record when these consultations are involved. Devotees of the treatment argue that individualized treatments are necessary for optimum results; I prefer to believe that the personal interaction with a caring practitioner produces a highly effective placebo response. Before you book an appointment, however, do ask yourself whether you're willing to pay big bucks for a placebo effect you might be able to harness via cheaper means, such as hydrotherapy.

Magnets

People who use magnets to relieve their pain tend to become magnet evangelists, exhorting friends and family, "You've just got to try these

DO-IT-YOURSELF HOMEOPATHY?

Although homeopathy is a controversial therapy with very little science standing behind it, the homeopathic remedies available for sale over the counter are cheap and apparently quite safe. Of the more than 450 remedies available, here are some of the most popular for back and neck pain, along with the symptoms they supposedly target:

Actaea racemosa or *Cimicifuga* for neck and upper-back stiffness
  and pain
Aesculus for pain low on the back, close to the tailbone
Arnica oil or gel for soft-tissue injury
Bellis perennis for deep-muscle injuries
Bryonia for severe back pain
Calcarea carbonica for back pain in overweight people
Rhus toxicodendron for neck pain
Ruta graveolens for back stiffness
Sulfur for back pain

things!" The folks at the health store may tell you that magnets work by stimulating nerve endings or by acting on the blood vessels, dilating them and increasing their capacity to carry oxygen. Does this enthusiasm have any basis in fact?

The studies say no. One well-controlled study looked at the effects of magnets on chronic low-back pain. Twenty patients were given either a bipolar magnet (which is arranged so that the poles alternate between north and south) or a look-alike fake strapped around their lower back. They wore them for six hours a day for three days out of a week. Then the groups switched, so the magnet group now had the sham treatment and the group that originally had the fake received the real thing. Again, they wore the magnets for three days over the course of a week. At the end of the experiment, patients ranked their pain on a scale of zero (no pain) to ten (the worst possible pain). Neither the sham magnets nor the real ones had any effect.

Of course, magnets can't do you much harm, either. If you want to try them, that's fine—as long as you buy an inexpensive product with a strength somewhere between 250 and 500 gauss. Don't use magnets if you have a pacemaker or an implanted defibrillator or spend time near someone who does. The magnetic field could affect the function of those crucial devices.

DO NOT USE THESE ALTERNATIVE TREATMENTS
FOR BACK AND NECK PAIN

Chiropractic Manipulation (for Neck Pain)

Although it's fine to try chiropractic manipulation for back pain, those of you who suffer from neck pain will have to try another therapy. Manipulation of the cervical spine (neck) is associated with a one-in-a-million risk of stroke. You don't want to be the "one" in that statistic.

Devil's Claw (Harpagophytum procumbens)

For hundreds of years, people indigenous to Africa's Kalahari Desert have used devil's claw to treat a variety of complaints. That long and exotic history is enough to attract a legion of followers here in the United States. But as a skeptical consumer, *you* want to know: does this herb have anything going for it but tradition?

Only one decent study has looked at devil's claw for back pain. This study, published by the *European Journal of Anaesthesiology,* examined a proprietary extract of devil's claw called Doloteffin. Two hundred patients with hip, knee, and back pain were given two tablets of Doloteffin per day for eight weeks. Then came the thoroughly impressive result: an improvement of 50 to 70 percent. The study's chief investigator hypothesized that devil's claw inhibits substances called cytokines, which regulate immune and inflammatory functions. Unfortunately, this study is missing a crucial element: a control group that would have allowed the investigators to compare Doloteffin to a placebo. Until there are higher-quality studies, I would not recommend devil's claw or Doloteffin.

The Complete Prescription for Controlling Chronic Back Pain

MAINTENANCE

Cardiovascular exercise: 30 minutes, at least 5 days a week

Specialized stretches and strength exercises: as recommended by a physical therapist or other expert, 3 days per week

Acetaminophen or NSAIDs: as needed; take no more than amount recommended on the label.

PENS: as needed

TO MANAGE EPISODES OF ACUTE BACK PAIN

Acetaminophen or NSAIDs: as needed; take no more than the amount recommended on the label.

Massage (for muscle spasms that accompany back pain): as needed

Hydrotherapy (for muscle spasms that accompany back pain): as needed

Keep moving to the extent possible; no heavy-duty activity

Heat wraps: as needed

The Complete Prescription for Controlling Chronic Neck Pain

MAINTENANCE

Cardiovascular exercise: 30 minutes daily, at least 5 days a week

Specialized stretches and strength exercises: as recommended by a physical therapist or other expert, 3 days a week

Acetaminophen or NSAIDs: as needed; take no more than the amount recommended on the label.

TO MANAGE EPISODES OF ACUTE NECK PAIN

Massage: as needed (no shiatsu massage)

Hydrotherapy: as needed

4

Satisfying Sleep

What Your Doctor Hasn't Told You About Alternative Medicine for Insomnia	And What the Health-Store Clerk Doesn't Know
Alternative medicine offers the hands-down best treatment for insomnia.	But it's not a pricey supplement.
Most over-the-counter sleep aids will leave you drowsy in the morning.	How some of the newer sleeping pills can break the insomnia cycle
In specific circumstances, melatonin has been proven to improve sleep.	Why you shouldn't use melatonin for long periods of time
Light therapy appears to be an effective sleep inducer.	Just how much light—whether from the sun or a light box—your body requires for good sleep
	(continued)

What Your Doctor Hasn't Told You About Alternative Medicine for Insomnia	And What the Health-Store Clerk Doesn't Know
When you need help falling asleep at night, it's reasonable to try valerian.	Certain other sleep-aid herbs can be dangerous.
You'll find much more information about these therapies—as well as many others—in the rest of this chapter.	

Sleep-onset insomnia (difficulty falling asleep at night) is an equal-opportunity disorder: it can strike at any age. But as you get older—and by "older" I mean 40 or 50—the odds of developing other sleep problems are stacked against you. You may awaken more easily in the middle of the night and find it more challenging to get back to sleep. Most of us in midlife and beyond spend more time in bed than we used to, and we still get less slumber. Your body's internal clock isn't the exquisite timepiece it once was and may now go off earlier than it used to, leaving you wide-eyed long before your alarm sounds. Menopause, with its notorious night sweats, can also cause frequent night wakings. And as you age, you spend less time in sleep's deeper stages.

Of course, there is tremendous variation among individual people and their sleep patterns. I have little trouble sleeping, but my wife struggles to get her nightly z's. Why the difference? No one is sure. Sleep success can also vary according to what's going on in your life. New baby, new job, new love, new challenges—all these can cause your normally good sleep to go bad. If your sleep was not that great to begin with, even a little stress can snowball into significant sleep losses. No matter what your sleep complaint—whether you can't nod off at bedtime or whether you have trouble sleeping through the night—this chapter will show you ways to improve your chances of getting truly restful sleep.

I want you to learn how to manage your sleep problems, because a good night's sleep is the key to a healthy life and successful aging. Deep sleep is especially vital. During deep sleep, your body secretes human growth hormone (HGH), which staves off fat accumulation and helps build strong bones and muscles. Scientists believe that another function of sleep is the consolidation of memories. Make sleeplessness a habit, and you might find yourself habitually forgetting where you placed your keys. Even worse, your body reacts to sleep deprivation as it does to other forms of serious stress—by releasing hormones like cortisol and adrenaline. Over time, those hormones can deplete your immune system and leave you more vulnerable to every kind of illness, from colds to cancer.

Lesser consequences of sleeplessness include difficulty concentrating, low energy, memory slips, irritability, and mood changes. Actually, it's hard to delineate whether mood problems like depression cause sleeplessness or insomnia causes the depression in the first place. Both are probably true, and it's likely they perpetuate a downward spiral of worsening symptoms.

I'm not telling you about the dire consequences of sleeplessness in order to frighten you. I certainly don't want you lose sleep over them! But if you have sleep problems, you need to take them seriously enough to get help. And contrary to what you might have heard, real help is out there. An intelligent combination of home-care techniques, alternative

IS YOUR BODY AGING . . . OR JUST VERY, VERY SLEEPY?

If your once-muscular middle has turned to flab, or if you're finding it harder to remember the names of your kids' teachers, or if you take to bed with colds and flus more frequently than you used to, don't assume that you're suffering the inevitable effects of aging. Instead, you may be feeling the consequences of accumulated sleep loss. Read this chapter for ways to pay off your sleep debt and start cashing in on better health.

therapies, and the occasional prescription sleeping pill can help most people learn to love bedtime again, not dread it. Even if you suffer from a seemingly die-hard case of insomnia, alternative medicine offers you an excellent strategy for better-quality sleep.

Better Sleep Begins at Home

When doctors exhort you to "make sleep a priority," what do they mean? Quit your demanding, twelve-hour-a-day job? Ignore your sick children who wake crying at 2 A.M.?

I have major career commitments and young children, and I'd never sacrifice either one of them to get more sleep. Yet I've always made sleep that proverbial "high priority." As I've grown older and found sleep more elusive, I've taken aggressive steps to make sure I get my much-needed eight hours. That way, I wake up ready to face the challenges of job and family with a good disposition and sense of humor.

Here are seven easy ways to maximize sleep time:

1. *Start with your mattress and pillow.* Mattress salespeople love to tell prospective buyers that although high-quality mattresses cost about an extra quarter per night you sleep on them, they'll pay for themselves in your improved efficiency at work the next day. They're right. Invest the time and money necessary to get a mattress and pillow that are comfortable and right for your sleep needs.

2. *Make sure your bedroom is lightproofed and soundproofed.* Light and sound are powerful sleep disrupters. Hang drapes (not just blinds) over your windows to make your room both quieter and darker. Try blackout drapes if necessary. Check for internal lights and noises as well. Do you have a clock radio with a bright digital display that aims a beacon of light toward your

pillow? Turn the display away from your eyes when you're ready to sleep. If nighttime noises are a problem, purchase a machine that neutralizes sound.

3. *Get active.* As shown by study after study, cardiovascular exercise is one of the best ways to ensure high-quality sleep. When I spend part of the day playing golf or tennis, I know that I will get a good sleep that night. I recommend 30 minutes of cardiovascular exercise daily.

4. *Get outside.* The combination of sunlight and fresh air is like a sleeping tonic. I love sailing, and I do not remember a day spent aboard a boat that was not followed by passing out shortly after my head hit the pillow. Of course, taking a day off to sail or hike or just enjoy the weather isn't always possible (and you should always be careful not to overdo sun exposure if you're not wearing sunscreen). As you'll read later in the chapter, exposing yourself to bright light indoors is the next best thing to being outdoors.

5. *Relax.* The bedtime ritual of taking a mental spin down your worry list is completely counterproductive. I know it's hard to break a lifelong habit of worrying at bedtime, but try setting aside another time of day for thinking about the things that bother you. How about doing your prime worrying as you take a walk or ride a bike? That way, you can work up a head of mental steam—and then blow it off as you work out. Or write down all your problems or things to do a few hours before bedtime. Then you won't have to stay awake worrying that you won't remember what to worry about tomorrow! If these strategies don't work, try using whatever method of relaxation you most enjoy. You can find more information about relaxation therapies later in this chapter.

6. *Avoid caffeine.* You probably know to avoid coffee and black tea before bed, but there are other foods and drinks that contain

enough caffeine to keep you awake: chocolate, most green teas, and colas and other sodas, like Mountain Dew. People have varying levels of sensitivity to caffeine. Some can't get near caffeine after noon, whereas others can enjoy a coffee and piece of chocolate just before bed without any effects on sleep at all.

7. *Avoid alcohol before bedtime.* Again, you need to understand your own sensitivity. Alcohol actually sends me off to sleep faster than usual and has no ill effects except an occasional trip to the bathroom (it's a diuretic). But most people find that although alcohol may help them drift off, they wake up, fully stimulated, three or four hours later. Find out which group you belong to—mine, or the majority—and drink accordingly.

SLEEP LESS, LIVE LONGER?

My ears are still ringing from the loud media buzz regarding a study at the University of California, San Diego, claiming that people who sleep more than seven hours a night have shorter lives than their wakeful counterparts. What was often lost in the news cycle was that there are many other well-conducted studies proving exactly the opposite. The fact remains that each of us has an ideal sleep time. I need eight hours of sleep to feel my best. Others might need as few as five or as many as ten. Unless you log in your ideal number of hours, you're playing fast and loose with your health.

How much sleep do you need to operate most efficiently and pleasurably during the day? Here's how to find out:

- Go to bed 15 minutes earlier than your usual bedtime and wake up at your normal time. The next day, gauge your response. Are you less tired? More alert? Do you generally feel better? If so,

(continued)

add another 15 minutes of sleep the next night. Keep going until you find a bedtime that leaves you feeling great the entire day that follows. That's your optimum bedtime.

- If you are wondering if you need *less* sleep, go to bed 15 minutes later than your usual bedtime, and wake up at the same time the next day. If you experience no difference in alertness or level of fatigue, try cutting back by another 15 minutes each night until you discover the right amount of sleep for you.

Conventional Medicine for Sleeping Problems

So what about sleep medications? Many people think of them as an addictive trap: take one and you're hooked for life. Sleeping pills got their bad reputation in the days when Betty Ford announced her fight with addiction to tranquilizers, and *Valley of the Dolls,* starring Hollywood women and their favorite sedatives, was a box-office hit. Back then, the sleeping pill of choice was nearly always a barbiturate. Today we know that this class of drugs leads to physical addiction; fortunately, now there are much better medications available.

The latest prescription drugs for sleep do not appear to be physically addicting. Some of the newest sleep aids, including zaleplon (Sonata), are short-acting drugs, meaning that they don't remain in your system very long—so you won't stagger through the next morning in a stupor. It's no surprise that most people prefer these medications. Normally good sleepers who are suffering from transient insomnia can get six to eight hours of sleep out of a dose, but some chronic insomniacs will find that these drugs last only three or four hours. For people who wake up early in the morning, that's not such a bad thing. Instead of taking the drug at bedtime, they can take a dose when they wake up at 3 A.M. The medicine will send them off to sleep for three or four hours, so that they arise at a more normal hour, alert enough to solve the crossword puzzle in morning paper. An intermediate-acting sleep medication, such as zolpidem (Ambien), may also be helpful.

If you've suffered a bad experience with sleep medications, it's possible you were taking long-acting medications that hang around your system for quite a while. These medications—including estazolam (ProSom), flurazepam (Dalmane), and quazepam (Doral)—can produce withdrawal symptoms and pack the knockout punch of barbiturates, carting you off to eight hours of slumber and then dumping you unceremoniously into a long, groggy wake-up period that can last half the day. They are drugs you should avoid, with one exception: the popular new sleep medication eszopiclone (Lunesta), which should leave you with less of a drug hangover.

Another drug, ramelteon (Rozerem), is in an entirely different drug category. It acts in a manner similar to melatonin—which is discussed later in this chapter—and works well for people who have trouble getting to sleep at bedtime.

Although it's tempting to believe that over-the-counter sleeping pills are gentler than prescription medications, watch out. Almost all over-the-counter sleep aids contain diphenhydramine (Benadryl), a potent antihistamine that lingers in your body a very long time. After taking these pills, many of us get a diphenhydramine hangover and can barely keep our eyes open the next day. If you drive to work, that's a dangerous disadvantage. These pills can also cause blurred vision, prostate problems, dizziness, delirium, and dementia. I probably don't need to tell you to stay away from these medications.

Although neither the long-acting or short-acting new drugs are physically addicting, it's possible that their continual use will lead to psychological addiction—meaning that you'll start to believe you can't get to sleep without your little white pill. Soon enough, that kind of doubt becomes a self-fulfilling prophecy. That's why all sleep medications are best reserved to pull you through the occasional rough patch. But during times of great stress when you're up for nights on end, don't hesitate to make smart use of sleep medications.

The Discriminating Consumer's Guide to Insomnia Alternatives

Conventional sleeping pills work, but only as a stopgap measure. How about more natural sleep aids? Alternative medicine provides a wide variety of options with a correspondingly wide variety of results. One therapy in particular—cognitive-behavioral therapy—appears to be the Holy Grail of insomnia research: a long-term solution for the chronically sleep-deprived.

HIGHLY RECOMMENDED ALTERNATIVE TREATMENTS FOR SLEEP PROBLEMS

Cognitive-Behavioral Therapy

Would it shock you to learn that the most effective sleep aid is not a pill? Cognitive-behavioral therapy (CBT) is probably the closest thing we have to a cure for insomnia. CBT is a short-term, highly effective form of psychotherapy that can be applied to a wide variety of health problems. When it's used for sleep, CBT doesn't try to adjust your chemistry with nightly pills. Instead, a CBT specialist can help you develop a plan that adjusts your sleep behavior.

Chronic insomnia is such a frustrating and apparently intractable problem that it can be hard to convince people that CBT, in all its simplicity, really works. But my examination of more than fifty studies involving more than 2,000 patients convinced me that in patients with chronic insomnia, behavioral interventions (which are all part of CBT) are the way to go. Their success rate is stellar compared with that of most other sleep therapies, running higher than 50 percent. (They are also ter-rific for those of us who suffer from occasional sleeplessness.) After a few weeks of treatment, the time it takes to get to sleep and the time it takes to return to sleep after awakening improve to nearly normal levels. Best of all, the effects are long-lasting, handing CBT a hefty advantage over drugs or herbs that may work for only one night at a time.

One of the best behavioral techniques for reducing insomnia is called stimulus control, and it asks you to restrict certain types of sleep behaviors. That may sound counterproductive, but it's not as grueling as you may think. Here's a breakdown of its steps. It can be reassuring to the have the guidance of a CBT specialist, but you can also try these on your own:

1. Establish a standard wake-up time for each morning. No sleep-ing in on weekends or after sleepless nights!

2. Use the bed and bedroom only for sleep. Keep the television, computer, work desk, and other stimulating objects out of the bedroom. You want to associate the bedroom with sleep, not *The Late Show.*

3. Anytime you are awake at night for more than 15 minutes, get out of bed. Go to another room, turn on the light, and perform a quiet activity like reading, knitting, listening to books on tape, or writing letters. Avoid the television, which can rouse you to wakefulness—unless you are like me and TV puts you to sleep. (I guess it depends on the show.) Return to bed only when you feel sleepy, once again giving yourself 15 minutes to fall asleep. No matter how tired you are, wake up at your scheduled time the next morning.

4. Do not nap during the day, even if you are very sleepy. Obvi-ously, do not try to drive long distances or operate heavy equip-ment when you are exhausted.

5. Learn a relaxation technique to loosen those tense muscles and speed you off to dreamland.

Keep this up for at least four weeks to see improvements, although many of you with temporary insomnia will see results much faster.

The purpose of any cognitive-behavioral treatment is to alter your sleep habits and behaviors. Sleep restriction aims to break any association of bed and the bedroom with wakefulness and then teach your mind and body to connect being in bed solely with being asleep. In addition to sleep restriction, CBT includes correction of any misperceptions about sleep requirements and the effects of sleep on daily function. CBT patients are also taught to practice the elements of good sleep hygiene (avoidance of caffeine as necessary, reduction of light and sound disturbances, and so on) that I have described earlier.

Cognitive-behavioral therapy was tested in a controlled study conducted at Duke University Medical Center. The investigators asked 75 subjects to participate in CBT, progressive muscle relaxation alone, or a placebo behavior therapy. Each group was treated for six weeks. Six months later, the researchers checked back in with their subjects.

The results were astonishing. The CBT group reduced the amount of sleep fragmentation—the number of night awakenings and time taken to get back to sleep—by nearly 50 percent. The other groups experienced only limited success, reducing sleep fragmentation by 16 percent in the relaxation group and 12 percent in the placebo group.

An even more compelling reason to try CBT is its long-term success rate. A study at the Medical College of Virginia/Virginia Commonwealth University enrolled insomniacs who had experienced difficulty going to sleep for at least six months and who suffered poor functioning, fatigue, or mood disturbance during the day. Seventy-eight patients were chosen and randomly selected to receive one of four treatments: sleep medication with temazepam (Restoril, a long-action prescription sleep aid), CBT, a combination of temazepam and CBT, or a placebo.

The results? After eight weeks of treatment, both CBT and drugs had worked, with the combination of CBT and drugs having the most potency. Things changed when researchers followed up with their patients at three, twelve, and twenty-four months. With each check-in, the CBT group held on to its good sleep while the drug groups gradually began to show signs of sleep loss. By twenty-four months, all subjects who were treated with drugs were relapsing into their initial pattern of sleep problems—but the CBT group had maintained its improvement.

Sleep experts were excited by this study because it focused on patients over 65 years of age and showed that sleep loss in this notoriously sleep-deprived age group can be successfully treated. A study at the Beth Israel Deaconess Medical Center in Boston showed that CBT is the best treatment for insomnia in younger patients as well.

If you have insomnia that isn't resolved after a few nights, try CBT. It works for those of you who grind your teeth through late nights as well as those who rise earlier than you wish. It's also drug-free and inexpensive.

Light Therapy

Most of us have at least one thing in common with the late John Denver: sunshine on our shoulders (or anywhere else) makes us happy. But diminished mobility or confinement to a nursing home too often means that elderly Americans are deprived of this simple pleasure. So are younger people who live in northern latitudes or work from dawn till dusk in windowless offices. Can our nationwide lack of sleep be caused by a lack of light?

Although it's not advisable to expose yourself to strong sunlight for long periods, there's a good biological reason we enjoy catching a few rays. Exposure to light during the day encourages nighttime release of melatonin, helping your body sleep and wake in appropriate cycles.

In an Australian study, 33 older adults wore light-exposure meters on their clothing and movement detectors on their wrists as they went about their normal activities. The Australian scientists found a significant relationship between light exposure and daytime activity and quality of sleep. The subjects whose daily routines exposed them to 3000 lux (moderately bright light) were far more likely to enjoy a good night's sleep, with fewer night awakenings. The average American gets only 500 lux a day, and nursing-home patients receive a dismal 50 lux daily. Is it surprising that nursing-home residents have the worst sleep problems of any of us?

There are plenty of ways to get your daily dose of light. Get outside into sunlight as much as possible. Be sure to put on sunscreen to protect your skin from ultraviolet light. (Sunscreen does not block sunlight's effect on your sleep.) If you can't get outside, work and play in a brightly lit area. If that is impossible, buy a light box—which is literally a box containing high-intensity lightbulbs that mimic the effects of natural sunlight—and put it next to your desk or place of work. Set it for at least 3000 lux and use it for 30 minutes a day. Light boxes are readily available online and at specialty stores.

If you tend to fall asleep early and awaken early, get your light—whether from the sun or a box—as late in the day as possible. Conversely, if you can't get to bed until late at night, try to get sun exposure in the morning.

Relaxation Therapies

"Just relax!" is advice commonly given to people with sleep problems. That's easier said than done, especially if you're in the habit of chewing over the day's problems in bed, or if the fear of yet another sleepless night makes you anxious. When you can't will yourself to "just relax," consider these techniques for quieting your mind:

PROGRESSIVE MUSCLE RELAXATION. Over and over, studies show that this easy technique reduces the amount of time it takes to fall asleep—and to get back to sleep after waking too early. Here's how to do it: Lie on your back and spend a few moments breathing deeply. Then concentrate on relaxing the different regions of your body, starting with your toes, moving up to your feet, and so on until you end by releasing the muscles of your neck, jaw, and face. It can help to imagine that your muscles are slowly melting. For some people, tensing the groups of muscles before relaxing them makes this process easier.

MEDITATION. You may think of meditation as something to do while you're wide awake, but three well-controlled studies show that this ancient technique can help you drift off to sleep more quickly. Meditation as defined by these studies is very similar to the relaxation response, in which you use repeated words, images, or activities to induce an enjoyable state of mental calm. If you'd like to try engaging your relaxation response, see the instructions on pages 19 and 20—though obviously you'll want to choose the quieter forms (such as a silently repeating a word) over the more active ones (such focusing on arm motions while swimming) for this purpose.

GUIDED IMAGERY. Mentally place yourself into a relaxing or neutral setting. I like to imagine that I'm in a dark elevator, going downward—and feeling my body getting heavier and more relaxed floor by floor.

BIOFEEDBACK. By helping you understand how your body responds to stress—and then showing you how to control those stress responses—biofeedback can reduce the time it takes you to get to sleep. It isn't any more effective than other relaxation methods, however. As biofeedback is both expensive (if your insurance carrier doesn't pay for it) and time-consuming, try this only when progressive muscle relaxation, meditation, and imagery have failed.

RECOMMENDED ALTERNATIVE TREATMENTS
FOR SLEEP PROBLEMS

Melatonin

A few years ago, it seemed that any book with *melatonin* in the title rocketed toward best-sellerdom. Melatonin's proponents claimed that this hormone could cure insomnia and make you young again. Yes, the fountain of youth in a bottle! These claims were propelled by Italian investigators who reported that old mice that were given melatonin appeared more youthful. But these mice were unusual in that they were deficient in melatonin to begin with. When melatonin is given to normal mice and humans, there is no evidence that the aging process is arrested or slowed.

Despite my obvious skepticism toward books that describe melatonin—or any other pill—as a "miracle," it makes good sense to investigate melatonin as a natural sleep aid. That's because this hormone plays a key role in the normal human sleep/wake cycle. Melatonin release peaks between 8 and 10 P.M., just before most of us go to sleep.

Melatonin appears to be useful in several circumstances. First, it helps readjust the altered biological cycle of shift workers who frequently change from day schedules to night and back again. It's also good for resetting your biological clock when traveling across time zones or on a Sunday night after staying up late all weekend. Finally, blind people can use it to help them maintain a normal sleep/wake cycle.

Given these melatonin successes, it's tempting to conclude that melatonin could help those of us with garden-variety sleeping problems. But hormones are tricky chemicals that don't always perform according to our wishes or even our best scientific theories.

One of the best studies of melatonin took place in Oregon. In this controlled trial, 14 patients were given either immediate or delayed-release forms of melatonin or a placebo at different times in the night. Neither the patients nor the investigators knew who received which medication. As in many other studies, melatonin decreased the amount of time it took patients to fall asleep. Interestingly, it also reduced internal body temperature, which theoretically should improve slumber—but this theory was deflated when patients reported no changes in their overall quality or quantity of sleep. Even more disheartening, neither melatonin nor a placebo caused changes in sleep physiology, ability to return to sleep after awakening, or energy levels the following day. Other well-conducted trials have also shown that while melatonin may decrease the time between when you lay your head down and when you fall asleep, it doesn't change general sleep quality or improve other aspects of slumber. The response rate appears to be highly variable, working for a few lucky individuals but not for most.

Although the evidence for melatonin for general insomnia is luke-warm, it has no apparent side effects when taken for a limited period of time. If one of your chief complaints is difficulty falling asleep, you could certainly give melatonin a try. Just don't expect it to help you remain asleep through the night.

DOSAGE AND SIDE EFFECTS: The American Academy of Sleep Medicine does not recommend the use of melatonin without medical supervision—and in Europe, melatonin is available by prescription only. Be sure to talk with your doctor before using this supplement and follow his or her instructions. Evidence indicates that the best dose of melatonin is 3 milligrams of an extended-release formula taken an hour before bedtime.

Use melatonin only on an as-needed basis. We've all learned the hard way that other hormones (such as estrogen) that are reasonably safe in the short term carry surprising side effects when used for a long time. It's wise to assume that melatonin might surprise us with dangers of its own after months or years of use. Don't use melatonin if you take calcium channel blockers, amphetamines, isoniazid (used to treat tuberculosis), or other sedatives, including alcohol.

Most melatonin products are created from synthetic products, but some are made using the brain tissue of cows. In this case, natural definitely isn't better. The cow-based products put you at risk of bovine illnesses, possibly including the human form of mad cow disease, and could cause additional problems for people with allergies to cow proteins.

Hydrotherapy

There aren't many good studies of hydrotherapy—the use of water as a healing agent—for the treatment of insomnia. But good scientific logic indicates that a hot soak can help to send you to sleep because a drop in body temperature triggers your sleep response. (Admittedly, scientific logic doesn't always play out in real-life circumstances, as we've seen with melatonin.) The best way to achieve that temperature drop is to heat your body up and then let it cool down. So encourage the rise and fall of your temperature by taking a hot Jacuzzi or shower right before bed. Then turn down the thermostat in your bedroom and let nature take its course. Don't get into very hot water if you have a heart condition or any other medical condition for which heat is contraindicated.

ACCEPTABLE ALTERNATIVE THERAPIES FOR SLEEP PROBLEMS

Valerian (Valeriana officinalis)

If you wander into a health store and inquire about sleep remedies, you are almost certain to find yourself guided toward valerian. This herb has been used as a sleep aid for millennia and is recommended for sleep problems by Germany's Kommission E. Although no one knows exactly what constitutes valerian's active ingredients, the herb's potency is generally attributed to valeric acid.

Valerian exhibits a contrast between how scientists feel it should work and how it actually performs. Lab studies show that valerian can help people slip into the much-needed deep stages of sleep—but subjects in clinical trials don't find valerian of much practical use. A high-quality study in Australia involved 24 insomnia patients who were given either valerian or a placebo for a week. After a washout period of five days, the patients switched treatments. Valerian was not significantly better than placebo for getting to sleep, staying asleep, or feeling refreshed the next day.

In a kind of Battle of the Sleeping-Pill Stars, Canadian researchers pitted valerian against two other sleep aids: diphenhydramine (the ingredient found in over-the-counter sleeping pills) and Restoril (a prescription sleeping medication), as well as a placebo. Restoril took home a dubious double blue ribbon for the most sedation but also the greatest number of side effects, with diphenhydramine coming in second in both categories. Neither valerian nor the placebo caused impairment of function the following day—but they also failed to improve sleep.

So what should you do? Some people swear by valerian, while many others find it useless. But valerian has been used for decades in Europe and other countries with few reports of side effects. If you are having trouble getting to sleep, you can try valerian—and hope that you are one of the fortunate few who respond well to this herb.

DOSAGE AND SIDE EFFECTS: Take 300 to 500 milligrams of valerian extract one hour before bedtime. Alternatively, place one teaspoon of dried valerian in a teacup and pour boiling water over the herb. Steep the tea for 15 minutes and strain before drinking. Valerian can smell a bit like old socks, so you might want to mix your extract or tea with an assertively flavored juice; pineapple juice works well. Adverse effects are unusual with valerian, although reported side effects include headache, dizziness, palpitations, depression, and mild gastrointestinal upset. Use caution if you are also taking medications for anxiety or depression, and never take valerian with other sedatives or alcohol. If you are planning to undergo surgery, tell your physician if you are taking valerian, as it may interact with some of the sedatives used during surgical procedures. And if you take valerian for several nights in a row and then stop, you may experience withdrawal symptoms—which reinforces my recommendation that sleep medications, including herbal ones, should be taken only occasionally.

Acupuncture

Good news: most studies of acupuncture indicate that it is an effective therapy for insomnia. Bad news: these studies were poorly conducted and published in journals of less than stellar quality. Most of these trials were not performed with controls in place, although it's difficult to find a good placebo control for acupuncture. Significantly, when the National

Institutes of Health reviewed acupuncture, it did not list insomnia as an indication for its use.

Often I tell patients with a keen interest in acupuncture to go ahead and try it, even if it hasn't yet been proven to help their particular medical problem. People who are strongly attracted to acupuncture are most likely to reap the benefits of a placebo effect, and acupuncture is unlikely to cause side effects. But when there are such promising results for other alternatives, why invest the time and money?

Aromatherapy

The scent of English lavender is reputed to induce sleep. Although there is no good literature to support the use of this herb, it produces few side effects and is approved by Germany's Kommission E for sleep problems. If you enjoy tucking a lavender sachet under your pillow or infusing your bedroom with its fragrance, why not? Unless you are allergic to it, lavender will probably do no harm. But if you don't see results in a few days, it's time to try something else. Keep using lavender if you enjoy it, but add another sleep aid that really works for you.

DO NOT USE THESE ALTERNATIVE TREATMENTS
FOR SLEEP PROBLEMS

Kava kava (Piper methysticum)

This Polynesian herb has long been reputed to induce drowsiness and relax muscles, leading many people to try it as a sleep aid. Nevertheless, there is scant literature available on the kava connection to sleep. The exception is insomnia that's specifically related to anxiety—and there the evidence is inconclusive. (See chapter 5, "Taming Depression and Anxiety," for more information.) The one thing that's clear about kava kava is that it can have serious side effects, including liver failure. For that reason, I do not recommend kava under any circumstance.

The Complete Prescription for Satisfying Sleep

TO MAINTAIN GOOD SLEEP
Relaxation techniques: as needed
Cardiovascular exercise: 30 minutes daily
Light therapy: frequent exposure to sunlight, or 3000 lux exposure
　　for 30 minutes daily

FOR DIFFICULTY SLEEPING
The following can be used in addition to the techniques listed above.
Cognitive-behavioral therapy: use as needed for occasional sleepless-
　　ness; chronic insomniacs should plan to try it for at least four
　　weeks before getting the techniques down pat.
Hydrotherapy: Jacuzzi or hot bath/shower as needed
Valerian (for occasional sleep-onset problems): 300 to 600 milligrams
　　taken 1 hour before bedtime
Melatonin (for special circumstances as listed or for occasinal sleep-
　　onset problems): 3 milligrams of an extended-release formula
　　1 hour before bedtime (can be taken in conjunction with valerian)
Rozerem (ramelteon): for sleep-onset problems; take as prescribed.
Other prescription sleeping medications (Ambien, Sonata, Lunesta):
　　for occasional trouble sleeping when great stresses are present;
　　take as prescribed.

5

Taming Depression
and Anxiety

**WHAT YOUR DOCTOR HASN'T TOLD YOU
AND THE HEALTH-STORE CLERK DOESN'T KNOW
ABOUT ALTERNATIVE MEDICINE FOR
DEPRESSION AND ANXIETY**

What Your Doctor Hasn't Told You About Alternative Medicine for Depression and Anxiety	And What the Health-Store Clerk Doesn't Know
Saint-John's-wort may be an effective treatment for certain forms of depression.	The best strategies for getting a consistent dose
Fish oils and folic acid may improve mood.	In cases of severe depression, no supplement or herb is a substitute for medical treatment.
Insufficient exposure to sunlight can lead to depression.	How much light you need to ward off depression and how to get it
Sleep deprivation is a factor in many cases of anxiety and depression.	One of the most popular herbs for treating anxiety-related insomnia can cause liver damage.

(continued)

What Your Doctor Hasn't Told You About Alternative Medicine for Depression and Anxiety	And What the Health-Store Clerk Doesn't Know
Applied relaxation therapy is a gentle but effective treatment for anxiety.	It's also far superior to most herbs sold to relieve anxiety.
You'll find much more information about these therapies—and many others—in the rest of this chapter.	

In one national survey, nearly 10 percent of the respondents reported suffering from depression or anxiety. Many suffered from both: more than a third of people with anxiety were also depressed. In a strong indicator that people perceive conventional medicine as inadequate for mood disorders, the majority of sufferers had tried alternative medicine for their problems during the twelve months leading up to the survey.

Generalized anxiety disorder (GAD) often goes unrecognized for a lifetime, perhaps because some people dismiss the exaggerated worries and fears that characterize this disorder as silly or unimportant. Let me set things straight: generalized anxiety disorder is a real disease. Although its sufferers recognize that their fears are out of proportion to reality, they are unable to change their feelings, and experience continually high and damaging levels of stress. Other typical features of GAD include a heightened state of awareness and feeling constantly on edge, fatigue, difficulty concentrating, irritability, muscle tension, and insomnia. These symptoms distinguish GAD from the normal anxiety that occurs in response to trying circumstances (such as speaking in public or asking for a raise) and fades when those circumstances are over.

Depression is a separate condition, although as I noted above, it often teams up with anxiety in a double whammy of mood disorders. Some forms of depression are normal and predictable. If you lose a spouse, parent, child, or close friend, you will probably be depressed. If you lose your job, are turned down for a promotion, or are getting divorced or separated from your spouse, you may also feel depressed. This is situational depression and an appropriate reaction to difficult circumstances. In many cases, the depression will disappear with time and does not require treatment other than the support of friends and relatives and some well-chosen home-care strategies.

Depression that is not clearly linked to a troubling life event can be much more difficult to shake. Encounters with depression can take place anywhere along a wide spectrum of intensity. On one end is dysthymia. People with dysthymia may feel blue or out of spirits and experience low-level malaise, sleeping problems, or fatigue. This is a mild form of depression that responds well to lifestyle modifications as well as some herbs and other alternative treatments. At the far end of the spectrum is clinical depression, which features serious problems with sleep, loss of appetite, difficulty concentrating, and a sense of overwhelming helplessness and boredom. Clinical depression does more than make life miserable for its victims—it greatly increases the risk of many health problems, including heart disease. Throughout the world, depression is a leading cause of disability.

Severe depression and anxiety are deadly diseases that need immediate attention. Alternative medicines are not substitutes for psychiatric or pharmaceutical treatments for these problems, although some may be used in conjunction with professional help. If you are showing signs of serious depression or anxiety, put the herbs on hold and get the help you really need.

Conventional medicine offers effective treatment for anxiety and depression, but many people with mild to moderate depression choose to look elsewhere. They may feel philosophically opposed to taking psychoactive drugs—or they may love what the drugs do for their mood but hate the side effects on their bodies. If you belong to either group, you're in luck. There are plenty of alternatives that can calm your mind and brighten your outlook. The best of these are inexpensive or even free.

Conventional Medicine for Depression and Anxiety

The majority of Americans who suffer from clinical depression and GAD remain untreated. Why? One reason is the fear of taking medications for their condition. These fears aren't without grounds. Although psychopharmaceuticals have come a long way since the heyday of lithium and Thorazine, current drugs come with their fair share of side effects.

For people whose depression puts them at risk for serious consequences, antidepressant drugs make good sense. Many of these medications increase the availability of the neurotransmitters serotonin and norepinephrine, which help regulate mood. If you have a lesser form of depression, however, you may want to think twice before asking your doctor for a prescription. Even the latest generation of drugs (known as selective serotonin reuptake inhibitors, or SSRIs) can cause loss of libido, drowsiness, blurred vision, insomnia, weight gain, nausea, diarrhea, and tremors. These are not rare events. For example, one study found that 17 percent of people on SSRIs experienced sexual dysfunction. Other studies have found that as many as one-third of all women taking SSRIs are unable to achieve orgasm and that 50 percent of men on these drugs have problems ejaculating.

People with anxiety face a similar choice. Lexapro, a commonly prescribed antianxiety medication, works well—but some people can't tolerate the side effects (nausea, insomnia, ejaculation problems, and fatigue, among others) or just don't like the idea of altering their brain chemistry.

Psychoanalysis is another conventional approach to mood disorders, although it is fading in popularity. Insurance companies, who dislike the years-long treatment, have undoubtedly played a role in this phenomenon. But there's a better reason the rest of us are backing away from "talk therapy": there are no good studies proving its effectiveness.

Electroconvulsive therapy (ECT), once known as shock therapy, is making a comeback for the treatment of severe depression. This treatment, which induces seizure and can kill brain cells, is reserved only for those who do not respond to any other treatments.

At-Home Mood Elevators

There are some simple lifestyle changes that can help you respond to mood disorders. As I write this chapter, Los Angeles is experiencing the heaviest rainfall in decades. My spirits are suffering, probably because I'm missing out on the tennis and golf that provide me with two reliable mood elevators: aerobic exercise and sunlight.

Cardiovascular exercise is a wonderful way to prevent depression. Staying in shape makes you feel good about yourself and induces brain chemicals (such as endorphins, the body's natural feel-good hormones) that lift your mood. It also controls levels of stress hormones. When I turned 40, I had every reason to have a midlife crisis. I had left the National Institute on Aging to accept my dream job as director of a new research institute on aging in Denver. I had also met someone special. Then, within one week, the funding for the institute disappeared along with my new love. I had a definite case of situational depression and certainly qualified for a whopping midlife crisis. Fortunately, the mountains provided an unparalleled venue for exercise. As I began to bicycle up and down the Rockies, my brain was flooded with endorphins. I also played racquetball to release my frustration. One day, after mercilessly whipping my opponent (he was an exceptionally good sport), I took a shower. I vividly remember standing in the shower and thinking how good the water felt on my body. I said to myself, "If I can feel so good despite all the terrible things that are happening, then I will be okay!" and my situational depression melted away. I didn't realize it then, but I was taking one of the best possible antidotes—aerobic exercise—for mild to moderate depression and anxiety.

Sunlight can also be a solution. Spend a winter weekend in Alaska or

Scandinavia, where the sun may shine only one or two hours a day, and you'll appreciate the effects of sunlight on mood. Brain levels of serotonin take a dive during the dark winter months, which probably explains why seasonal depression is common in sunlight-deprived regions and why Scandinavian countries have some of the highest rates of suicide in the world. You don't need to live in an extreme latitude to experience the depressing effects of darkness—not if you're an American who drives to work with your headlights on and heads home after nightfall. If your depression tends to become worse in the winter, try spending more time every day by a sunny window. Better still, eat a healthful, quick lunch at your desk and then stroll around the block during your lunch break. (Sunlight deprivation is probably not a cause of anxiety, though getting extra light can alleviate insomnia, one of anxiety's sidekicks.)

If exposure to natural sunlight just isn't possible, light therapy can help. This treatment is described later in the chapter.

THE SLEEP/MOOD CYCLE

One of the main features of insomnia is depressed or anxious mood, and a frequent sign of depression and anxiety is an inability to sleep well. These problems tend to feed each other and trap you in a vicious cycle of sleeping less and feeling worse. If you suffer from sleeplessness in addition to depression or anxiety, you need to treat both problems. See chapter 4, "Satisfying Sleep," for ways to get a better night's rest.

The Discriminating Consumer's Guide to Depression and Anxiety Alternatives

For most cases of depression and anxiety, there is a host of gentle alternatives to pharmaceutical treatment. Because depression responds well to placebos, I suggest you seek out those therapies that you think are most likely to work for you. That way, your mind might give the healing process a boost.

If you suffer from severe depression or anxiety, you need to be under the care of a skilled psychiatrist—but alternative medicine can step in as a helpful adjunct. Be advised that certain supplements and herbs can mix dangerously with psychiatric medications.

HIGHLY RECOMMENDED ALTERNATIVE TREATMENTS FOR DEPRESSION AND ANXIETY

Cognitive-Behavioral Therapy

Cognitive-behavioral therapy (CBT) is a form of psychotherapy in which a counselor helps you identify distorted patterns of thought and habitual, counterproductive responses to difficult situations. You and the therapist then work together to find tools for taking greater control over life's stresses. CBT has been shown in several small clinical trials to be as effective as antidepressants and antianxiety medications in people with mild depression and anxiety. People with more stubborn mood disorders may consider using pharmaceuticals in addition to CBT, as the combination appears to have a synergistic effect. Your health-care provider will no doubt be happy to provide you with a referral to a good CBT expert.

CBT is usually a short-term treatment, but in the case of moderate to severe mood problems, plan on spending a year or two making weekly visits to the therapist. Fortunately, CBT is usually covered by insurance companies.

Applied Relaxation Therapy

As I've described, cognitive-behavioral therapy has been shown to work as well as drugs for mild mood disorders. If you suffer from mild anxiety, here's more good news: a mind-body therapy known as *applied relaxation therapy* has been shown to work as well as CBT.

Applied relaxation therapy bears a strong resemblance to guided imagery, another mind-body technique. In applied relaxation therapy, a patient is asked to think of a calming situation, perhaps floating on a raft in a gentle lake, or relaxing in the tall grass of a sunny meadow. The full imagining of every detail in the scenario—from the temperature of the lake water to the smell of the meadow flowers—relaxes both the muscles and the mind. The patient can then mentally return to this calm place during times of stress. For best results, ask your doctor for a referral to a therapist who is trained in applied relaxation therapy and can show you how to get the most from it.

Folic Acid

Folate, or folic acid—a B vitamin found in fruits and vegetables, beans, and grains—is a critical supplement for preventing heart attacks and colon cancer. It may also encourage the production of a chemical called S-adenosyl-L-methionine, which can boost serotonin levels.

The *Medical Journal of Australia* published a review of four double-blind, randomized, and controlled clinical studies of folic acid, and three of them found that when folic acid is combined with antidepressants, patients are more likely to improve than when they receive antidepressant therapy alone.

DOSAGE: Get 800 micrograms of folic acid daily from either food or supplements. For best results, use folic acid in combination with prescription antidepressants.

Light Therapy

Light therapy includes exposure to natural sunlight but is most associated with the use of light boxes. These are portable, lightweight boxes containing fluorescent tubes that mimic the quality of sunlight on a spring day. The use of light boxes may sound like a gimmick, but controlled studies show that it is effective against the kind of seasonal depression that flares up in the dark winter months. The therapy seems to work particularly well if the light is administered in the morning. If you suffer from seasonal depression, you might try undergoing just one hour of light therapy as a test. In one study, people who felt better after this minimal exposure went on to experience the best results with longer courses of light therapy.

In many nursing homes, the seasonless, sunless environment is a possible contributor to the high levels of depression among residents. When nursing-home residents were exposed to 10,000 lux of light from a light box for three hours every morning, their depression scores as measured on a standardized scale dropped substantially and actually approached the normal, nondepressed range. A lower level of light (3000 lux) did not produce a change in symptoms. To put these levels in perspective, most indoor light is equivalent to about 300 lux and intense sunshine can produce up to 100,000 lux.

It's not clear whether light therapy can help those whose depression is not linked to winter darkness or lack of sun. There have been studies indicating that bright light (5000 lux for two hours each morning) may be effective for nonseasonal depression, but this evidence is only preliminary. This therapy isn't useful for anxiety, though it can improve sleep.

If you suspect that your depression is connected to inadequate exposure to light, and if it's possible for you to get out in bright sunlight, do so. (Don't overdo your exposure, and wear sunscreen. Sunscreen will *not* block sunlight's beneficial effects on mood.) Should you require some extra assistance bringing light into your world, consider purchasing a light box (which can cost $200 to $500, but this is sometimes covered by insurance). You'll need one that produces 10,000 lux when it's set at a distance of two feet from your head. I recommend getting about 30 minutes of exposure daily.

RECOMMENDED ALTERNATIVE TREATMENTS
FOR DEPRESSION AND ANXIETY

Saint-John's-Wort (Hypericum perforatum)

Long before the term *miracle drug* came into use, people have ascribed miraculous or mystical qualities to Saint-John's-wort. Its botanical name can be traced to the phrase "over an apparition" and refers to an ancient belief that the odor of Saint-John's-wort was repellent to evil spirits and would make them fly away. Now there are many who believe that this herb can chase away the demons of depression. Is this also mere superstition? Apparently not, at least when it comes to mild forms of the disorder.

No one doubts that Saint-John's-wort has at least some effect on mood. It appears to work by increasing the level of several neurotransmitters, including serotonin and norepinephrine, along with dopamine, GABA, and L-glutamate. No other antidepressant—herbal or pharmaceutical—has such a wide spectrum of action. Its most potent ingredient is a chemical called hypericin, which acts similarly to antidepressants like Paxil, Prozac, and Zoloft. Other ingredients in Saint-John's-wort, including adhyperforin and hyperoside, may also help regulate brain chemicals. Saint-John's-wort also has far fewer side effects than antidepressant drugs.

People who respond the best to Saint-John's-wort appear to be those with mild depression. Out of 27 randomized, double-blind trials, 17 found Saint-John's-wort effective for mild to moderate depression, and 10 reported effects comparable with that of tricyclic antidepressants (a class of drugs that predates SSRIs).

Despite its chemical activity, Saint-John's-wort has turned in a lackluster performance for major depression. Very depressed patients who were given either Saint-John's-wort or a placebo for twenty-four weeks showed no difference in their responses.

The placebo effect throws a wrench into our full understanding of Saint-John's-wort. Placebos can improve depression symptoms so effectively that their performance sometimes rivals that of Zoloft and other proven pharmaceuticals. This could explain the difficulty in getting consistently positive results from Saint-John's-wort.

I do not recommend you try Saint-John's-wort if you have serious or even moderate depression. Your problem is too serious to allow experimentation with unproven herbs. Instead, talk to your doctor about using SSRIs or other prescription drugs. They have an excellent track record both in clinical practice and in well-controlled trials.

DOSAGE AND SIDE EFFECTS: If you suffer from dysthymia, or mild depression, it's reasonable to try Saint-John's-wort. It's difficult to obtain a consistent dose for Saint-John's-wort, as you can see from the box titled "What Are You Really Buying?" My advice is to find a product with at least 3 percent hyperforin and 0.2 percent hypericines. When the package runs out, buy the same product. This doesn't ensure consistency, but it's the best strategy you have. Start with one dose of 300 milligrams daily for three weeks. If symptoms persist, you can increase the dosage to 900 milligrams, divided into two or three daily doses.

Side effects for Saint-John's-wort include gastrointestinal upset, dry mouth, dizziness, constipation, and restlessness. Rarely, fair-skinned people will experience increased photosensitivity. Those with bipolar disorder must avoid Saint-John's-wort, because mania can sometimes occur. Since Saint-John's-wort increases serotonin levels in much the same way as SSRI drugs, it should not be taken with them. Saint-John's-wort can also interact with HIV drugs, cyclosporin, warfarin, digoxin, theophylline, anticonvulsants, oral contraceptives, and triptans. In one alarming report, two patients' bodies rejected their heart transplants because Saint-John's-wort reduced the effectiveness of cyclosporine, an immunosuppressive medication given to transplant recipients.

WHAT ARE YOU *REALLY* BUYING?

Several years ago, the *Los Angeles Times* sent bottles of Saint-John's-wort from ten different manufacturers to a laboratory to measure the amount of hypericin (the herb's most potent ingredient). The newspaper found that levels of hypericin varied significantly from the amount stated on the labels. When the herb manufacturers complained about the report, the *Times* sent the products to a second laboratory and came back with very similar results.

This inconsistency isn't unusual for herbal remedies, but it may be an even greater problem for Saint-John's-wort. When it became a popular treatment for depression, the price of this herb's flowers and leaves—which contain the active ingredients—shot up a hundredfold. Manufacturers may have been tempted to dilute their products with the inactive components of the herb, including stems and roots. As always with herbal products, "buyer beware" is the rule.

Fish oils (omega-3 fatty acids)

Fish oils that contain omega-3 fatty acids are best known for their beneficial effects on blood vessels, but you'll also hear claims that they elevate mood. Unfortunately, only one study has compared fish oil's effects on depression with those of a placebo—and the result was a tie between the two. But studies of fish oils used in conjunction with antidepressants have been much more encouraging. In one trial, patients who combined antidepressants with 1 gram of EPA (eicosapentaenoic acid) per day cut their depression scores in half.

More studies of fish oils are needed, but it's possible to draw practical conclusions from the available evidence. It makes sense to try them, especially in combination with pharmaceutical antidepressants.

DOSAGE AND SIDE EFFECTS: I recommend you use the same dosage that's necessary for good heart health. That's one to two servings of fatty fish (mackerel, herring, salmon, and tuna are good choices) per week or 1 gram daily of fish-oil supplements that contain EPA and DHA (docosahexanoic acid). Do not consume more than two servings per week of fatty fish, as many contain significant levels of mercury or other contaminants. Synthetic fish oils may be superior, although their side effects can include a fishy smell on the breath as well as gastrointestinal upset and bleeding.

Massage

Massage can lift your spirits. Can it also lift the cloud of mood disorders?

You might guess that a relaxing technique like massage can soothe anxiety, and studies appear to back that intuition up. Eight out of ten clinical trials have shown massage therapy to reduce anxiety and tension.

Only two trials meeting basic scientific criteria have been conducted on massage and depression, and both of those studies focused on children and adolescents. In the first study, depressed children and teens spent five days either receiving massage or watching relaxing videotapes. The second study looked at depressed teenaged mothers who were given either massage therapy or relaxation therapy over a five-week period. In both studies, the massage group showed a greater improvement.

These studies aren't conclusive, but they do indicate that massage may produce a short-term improvement for depression. We'll need more evidence before drawing stronger conclusions, especially for the long-range benefits of massage. Until then, it still makes good sense to enjoy a relaxing massage if it makes you feel better and you don't mind spending the money. Even if it doesn't directly affect your mood, massage might relax the tightened muscles that are the frequent companions of depression (as well as anxiety).

Yoga

As an antianxiety therapy, yoga remains unproven by good clinical trials. But there remains a lot to like about this therapy, which incorporates physical exercise, breath control, and relaxation techniques. Try a yoga class or two. At the very least, your tense muscles will feel looser and more limber afterward. Just be sure to sign up for a course that's appropriate for your level of experience and fitness. If you're a beginner, admit it. Finding yourself in an advanced class full of human pretzels (when you feel more like a stick) will just add to your stress.

ACCEPTABLE ALTERNATIVE TREATMENTS
FOR DEPRESSION AND ANXIETY

Acupuncture

Acupuncture's advocates claim that depression is caused when the yin and yang forces in the body are out of kilter. By restoring the proper balance between these forces, acupuncture can supposedly relieve depression. Westerners who find these concepts too mystical for their taste may appreciate a different theory regarding acupuncture's possible effects on depression: research on animals indicates that acupuncture can increase levels of the neurotransmitters norepinephrine and serotonin.

If you talk to alternative-medicine enthusiasts, you may hear about studies that have supposedly shown electroacupuncture (in which light electrical stimulation is applied to the needles) to be as effective as some pharmaceutical antidepressants. I do not place my faith in these studies, which were performed in China—where studies of acupuncture yield positive results with unsettling frequency—and included patients with several different forms of depression. Both of these factors make the results difficult to interpret.

More interesting are two Western trials that were small but used better standards and controls. In the first, acupuncture improved symptoms of depression, but no more than a placebo did. In the second, traditional acupuncture was more effective than the placebo, but the group showed only slighter better results than the one that received no treatment at all.

The jury's still out on acupuncture and depression, and I hope to see more studies in the future. Although it's too soon to come to a clear scientific pronouncement on this subject, acupuncture remains a safe therapy. If you wish to try it and don't mind the expense, go ahead.

Chamomile

Chamomile tea is a traditional folk prescription for anxiety. If you enjoy relaxing with a hot cup, that's great—put your feet up, inhale the sweet aroma, and sip away. But as there are no good studies of chamomile's supposed calming effects, don't make this herb your sole source of anxiety relief. Do not use chamomile if you have hay fever (an allergy to ragweed).

Valerian (Valeriana officinalis)

Valerian has long been used to help sleep problems. Today you may see it recommended for anxiety as well, perhaps because of the association between this disorder and insomnia. However, studies of valerian either show no effect for anxiety, or are very badly done, with few controls in place.

DOSAGE: Valerian has a long reputation as a safe herb with minimal side effects, but nevertheless I'd avoid taking it for anxiety—unless you are struggling with sleep problems. In that case, you can try the dosage suggested on page 96 and follow the instructions there. Be especially careful not to mix valerian with antianxiety medications, antidepressants, sedatives, or alcohol.

DO NOT USE THESE ALTERNATIVE TREATMENTS
FOR DEPRESSION AND ANXIETY

Kava Kava (Piper methysticum)

For centuries, Polynesian societies have enlisted the reputedly sedating effects of kava kava for use in their ceremonies. Now Americans and Europeans use it to relieve anxiety. Are they on to something? Kava kava contains chemicals called kavalactones, which appear to bind to neurochemicals like serotonin. It's not far-fetched to wonder if they might have an effect on mood.

However, it's too early to answer this question. In the only randomized, double-blind, placebo-controlled study of kava kava and anxiety, 37 patients with generalized anxiety disorder were given either kava kava or a placebo. While patients who received kava did better than those receiving placebo on certain anxiety measures, patients receiving the placebo did better on others.

More important than kava kava's effects on anxiety, however, are its effects on your liver. Eleven reported cases of liver failure following kava use have led health authorities in the United States, Germany, and Switzerland to issue warnings about this herb. Less alarming but more frequent side effects include skin scaling (although this usually occurs at doses of 400 milligrams of kavalactones, far above the usual dose of 100 to 200 milligrams).

5-HTP

5-HTP, an amino acid, may hold promise in the treatment of anxiety, especially in children, as well as depression. However, there is an unexplored downside to this treatment. 5-HTP is a relative of L-tryptophan, an effective sleep supplement that was used extensively in the 1970s and 1980s. But in 1989, an impurity inherent in the manufacturing of L-tryptophan led to deadly side effects. I don't recommend taking 5-HTP until the possibility of similar problems with this product is ruled out.

SAMe (S-adenosyl-L-methionine)

SAMe (S-adenosyl-L-methionine) is a chemical manufactured naturally in the body, and it plays a vital role in a number of critical metabolic processes. Because SAMe increases concentrations of dopamine and serotonin, two key neurotransmitters, there's been speculation that it can help alleviate depression.

In one study, patients suffering from both depression and Parkinson's disease cut their depression scores in half when given 800 to 3600 milligrams of SAMe. This study was small and did not use a control group or placebo, so its results are merely preliminary.

I advise holding off on SAMe until we know more about it. Not only do we lack solid evidence of its effectiveness for depression, it's extremely difficult to calibrate proper dosages. SAMe is absorbed so poorly through the intestine that many researchers give their subjects injectable SAMe, not the SAMe pills that are available at the health store. SAMe is also very unstable when exposed to air at room temperature, so it's unclear how much SAMe you'll get from the pills once you open the container and place it in your medicine cabinet.

SAMe also comes with the risk of diarrhea and other gastrointestinal side effects. It's particularly important for anyone with bipolar disorder to avoid SAMe, as the drug increases the risk of mania.

The Complete Prescription for Taming Depression and Anxiety

Note: If you have symptoms of severe depression or generalized anxiety disorder, seek professional help immediately; do not rely on alternative therapies alone.

Cardiovascular exercise: 30 minutes a day for a minimum of 5 days
a week

Cognitive-behavioral therapy: as prescribed by your doctor

Applied relaxation therapy: as desired

Fish oils: one to two servings of fatty fish per week or 1 gram daily
of fish-oil supplements that contain EPA and DHA

Folic acid: 800 micrograms daily from either food or supplements

Light therapy (for seasonal depression): 30 minutes of exposure daily
(3000 to 10,000 lux)

Massage: as needed for short-term improvement of symptoms

Saint-John's-wort (for dysthymia and mild depression only): start
with one dose daily, using 300 milligrams of a product containing
at least 3 percent hyperforin and 0.2 percent hypericines. If symptoms persist, increase to 900 milligrams daily, divided into two
or three doses across the day.

Yoga: as desired

Pharmaceutical antidepressants: as prescribed by your doctor

6

PMS:

Natural Symptom Relief

**WHAT YOUR DOCTOR HASN'T TOLD YOU
AND THE HEALTH-STORE CLERK DOESN'T KNOW
ABOUT ALTERNATIVE MEDICINE FOR PMS**

What Your Doctor Hasn't Told You About Alternative Medicine for PMS	And What the Health-Store Clerk Doesn't Know
Calcium is a highly effective source of PMS relief.	Which form of calcium is most efficiently absorbed into the body
Vitamin B$_6$ may reduce PMS symptoms.	Why it's all too easy—and dangerous—to overdose on this supplement
Evening primrose oil contains the omega-3 fatty acids that some PMS sufferers may lack.	Whether evening primrose oil actually has an effect on PMS symptoms
Chasteberry has been used for thousands of years to treat premenstrual distress.	How much proof stands behind this herb

You'll find much more information about these therapies—as well as many others—in the rest of this chapter.

During the menstrual cycle, there are major fluctuations in the amounts of female hormones in the bloodstream. These changes allow the uterus to thicken and engorge with blood, ensuring the ideal situation for fertilization and pregnancy. Unfortunately, hormonal fluctuations are also a recipe for the uncomfortable symptoms of premenstrual syndrome (PMS).

PMS symptoms usually occur in the six days preceding menstruation. They include water retention, mood changes, breast fullness, abdominal cramps, food cravings, headache, and fatigue. It's important to separate PMS, which affects 75 to 95 percent of women in their childbearing years, from a more severe condition called premenstrual dysphoric disorder (PMDD). PMDD affects only 3 to 8 percent of menstruating women and often isn't diagnosed until a woman is in her mid- to late 30s. This disorder includes a constellation of symptoms: depression, marked mood swings, irritability, anxiety, and sleep disturbances. These problems occur prior to menstruation but are relieved with the onset of bleeding.

Alt-med gurus are full of claims about the powers of one herb or another to treat PMS and PMDD. Many of these claims lack proof—but this doesn't mean you have to ignore *all* alternative medicine. Some of the best ways to relieve cramps, depression, water retention, and other PMS symptoms can be found in the supplement aisles.

Conventional Medicine for PMS: Effective . . . but with Side Effects

A wide range of pharmacological approaches has been used to treat the symptoms of PMS and PDD, including oral contraceptives and other hormonal therapies, NSAIDs, bromocriptine (for breast tenderness), and diuretic agents. If depression, mood instability, or sleep disturbances are present, antidepressants (especially Zoloft) may be prescribed. These drugs work well for many women, but all of them come with potential side effects: NSAIDs can cause gastrointestinal problems, bromocriptine may cause nausea, and antidepressants can lead to sexual dysfunction, insomnia, weight gain, and other problems.

Because of these side effects, many women seek alternative therapies that may be gentler. Some women tolerate conventional medicines quite well but view PMS as a naturally arising condition that calls for a natural and nonpharmaceutical approach to relief.

THE PMS/MENOPAUSE CONNECTION

Women who suffer from severe PMS are more likely to experience intense symptoms during menopause.

Get Moving!

If you're looking for the most natural way to lift your mood and bring down your discomfort, try going for a walk. You can also ride your bike, swim, or do anything else that gets your heart pumping. And you won't be alone: In a study of 1,800 women, more than half reported trying exercise to modify their PMS. A stunning 80 percent of this group felt that it worked! Women who exercised also showed better concentration, less pain, and brighter mood than those who didn't work out. I recommend getting at least 30 minutes of exercise a day, 5 days a week. Try to do this throughout the month, including those days when you feel cramping pains.

The Discriminating Consumer's Guide to PMS Alternatives

Heartening news for PMS sufferers: one of the best treatments for premenstrual syndrome is an inexpensive and safe supplement. If you have PDD, alternative medicine's bag of tricks holds something for you as well.

HIGHLY RECOMMENDED ALTERNATIVE TREATMENTS
FOR PMS

Calcium

Calcium is a highly effective alternative treatment for PMS. Among its many functions, estrogen regulates calcium metabolism and the absorption of calcium into the intestines. New scientific evidence shows that as estrogen levels wax and wane during the menstrual cycle, blood calcium levels also fluctuate. This is significant because having too little calcium (hypocalcemia) and too much calcium (hypercalcemia) are known to be associated with depression and anxiety, two of the most prominent PMS symptoms. It's been proposed that PMS is actually a form of temporary calcium deficiency.

In one excellent trial, nearly 500 women with PMS were given either 1200 milligrams of calcium carbonate or a placebo every day throughout three menstrual cycles. The women who used the placebo experienced symptom reduction of about 30 percent. But the women who took the calcium did even better, reporting a 48 percent reduction in depression and anxiety, as well as fewer problems with water retention, food cravings, and pain.

DOSAGE AND SIDE EFFECTS: Take 1200 milligrams of calcium daily for optimum relief of PMS symptoms. Calcium citrate is the best-absorbed form of calcium, though it can be pricey. If you need to watch your budget, you can try calcium carbonate instead. If you're taking prescription drugs or suffer from kidney stones, check with your doctor before taking any form of calcium.

To ensure that the calcium is properly absorbed into your body, you also need vitamin D. I prefer that you let your body trigger its own production of vitamin D by getting a little sunlight on your skin. You don't need much. Just 3 to 5 minutes in the sun (without sunscreen, and with your face and arms exposed) two or three times a week is enough. Try to avoid strong sunlight, particularly if you are fair-skinned, and certainly don't spend a lot of time in the full sun. If you live in a northern climate, the sun may not be strong enough during winter to help you manufacture vitamin D. You'll need to take 1000 IU of vitamin D per day during the colder months. Because overdoing the vitamin D can create toxic conditions in your body, make sure you take no more than those 1000 IU.

Light Therapy

There is some evidence that PMDD may be caused by disruptions to a woman's circadian clock. In one well-designed study, women with PMDD were randomly divided into two groups. One group received 30 minutes of light therapy each evening, using a light box that produced bright white light. Members of the second group were given a placebo: 30 minutes under a red fluorescent light. The group that received the bright white light had a significant reduction in depression and premenstrual tension when compared with either their previous condition or the placebo treatment.

This therapy appears to be a good choice for women with PMDD, but there are no trials yet of light therapy for PMS. Before buying a light box, you can try a free alternative: natural sunlight. Spend some time outside every day, or sit near a sunny window as you work. If that's not possible, look for light boxes in department stores and specialty shops and from online vendors. Be sure to purchase a box that produces 10,000 lux of bright white light. You'll need to sit near the light box for at least 30 minutes daily.

RECOMMENDED ALTERNATIVE TREATMENTS FOR PMS

Magnesium

Magnesium may be another smart supplement for PMS symptoms. This mineral fluctuates during the menstrual cycle, possibly affecting a woman's levels of serotonin and other neurotransmitters as well as biological factors. Three small but well-controlled trials have shown promising results for magnesium supplementation, varying from less fluid retention and headache to improved mood. Although I'd prefer to see larger studies of magnesium, there's no reason not to try moderate doses of this supplement now.

DOSAGE: Take 300 milligrams daily, and know that it may take up to two months before you see results. Most people experience no side effects from this dosage of magnesium, although a few develop mild diarrhea.

Chasteberry (Vitex agnus-castus)
(for breast pain and fullness only)

Chasteberry's Latin name is translated as "chaste lamb." Folklore has it that a concoction made from chasteberry seeds will reduce a person's sexual desire. We can only imagine what kind of sexist thinking might have caused the ancients to link this herb with women's health problems, but the fact remains that chasteberry fruit has been used for premenstrual problems for thousands of years. The question now is: What's the evidence?

There are active ingredients to be found in chasteberry fruit—such as flavonoids, antioxidants that combat the effects of free radicals. Perhaps these flavonoids account for the clinical finding that chasteberry appears to relieve some PMS symptoms, particularly breast pain and fullness. Short-term use yields fairly mild side effects. Some women experience nausea, allergy, diarrhea, weight gain, heartburn, increased menstrual bleeding, and stomach complaints. I'd like to see some long-term trials to more firmly establish chasteberry's safety and to compare chasteberry with standard medical treatment.

DOSAGE: Follow the dosage recommendations of Germany's Kommission E and try 30 to 40 milligrams by mouth daily—but take chasteberry for only a few months. If you are taking this herb for breast pain, make sure to see a doctor to rule out an underlying disorder. Because chasteberry might have an effect on female hormones, don't take it if you are breast-feeding (some breast-feeding mothers experience menstrual cycles).

ACCEPTABLE ALTERNATIVE TREATMENTS FOR PMS

Vitamin B_6

One study of vitamin B_6 supplementation in women with PMS concluded that this treatment reduced the severity of depressive and physical symptoms when compared with a placebo. Other studies, however, have shown no benefit to taking vitamin B_6. If this vitamin does have an effect on PMS, the means by which it does so are unclear. It's reasonable to try B_6 if you wish, but there are other, safer remedies for PMS.

DOSAGE: The promising study I cited above used a dosage of 50 to 100 milligrams daily, but you should stick with the lower dosage (50 milligrams). The Food and Nutrition Board of the Institute of Medicine has established an upper limit of 100 milligrams of B_6 per day for all adults. Excessive ingestion (2000 to 6000 milligrams) of B_6 can cause severe and permanent nerve damage. If you're taking a multivitamin that contains B_6 or eat fortified breakfast cereals, add up how much you're getting from these sources before adding even more B_6 in the form of a special supplement.

Cognitive-Behavioral Therapy (CBT)

Cognitive-behavioral therapy (CBT) is a practical and short-term form of psychotherapy. CBT's premise—which is that although you can't always control your pain, you can control your reactions to it—holds a certain amount of logic. But the available studies of CBT in connection with PMS are small and flawed. Most appear to show a terrific benefit for CBT but fail to measure the therapy against a good placebo. This problem makes it difficult to interpret the true results of the tests.

If CBT has piqued your interest (and if the cost is covered by your insurance provider), there's certainly no harm in trying it. And you just might discover a useful mental tool for managing your suffering.

Homeopathy

In one well-controlled study, 90 percent of women who received individualized homeopathic remedies reported a reduction in their PMS symptoms by 30 percent. (A 30 percent improvement might not sound like much, but it can mean the difference between being able to go to work and having to spend the day curled up against a heating pad.) A different trial, however, showed that 47 percent of women who received a *placebo* homeopathic remedy also reported an improvement in their PMS symptoms.

This large placebo effect makes it difficult to put homeopathy to a rigorous test. One possible explanation for the high placebo response is the intense one-on-one consultations homeopaths provide. This attentive give-and-take—not the chemically inert remedies—may itself stir the body's own healing mechanisms.

If you want to try homeopathy for PMS relief, do so with your eyes open. Individualized treatments of the kind studied above are safe, but they can be expensive. You can also try over-the-counter homeopathic remedies for PMS, such as *Pulsatilla*. These cost less than $10. But without the homeopathic consultation, you'll be less likely to engage a healing placebo response.

DO NOT USE THESE ALTERNATIVE TREATMENTS FOR PMS

Evening Primrose Oil (Oenothera biennis)

Evening primrose oil is a popular PMS treatment, thanks to a theory that women with PMS might have difficulty metabolizing omega-3 fatty acids (compounds that have protective effects on the heart and brain). Evening primrose oil is rich in omega-3 fatty acids, so some experts have wondered whether it could help reduce PMS symptoms. Clinical studies have not shown any significant effect on PMS, however. There's no reason to try it for this disorder.

AVOID THESE HERBS (FOR NOW)

Aside from chasteberry, you may hear of several other botanicals for PMS relief. Because none of them has been put through adequate clinical testing, I suggest you avoid the following herbs in favor of the PMS treatments that are known to work:

black haw (*Viburnum prunifolium*)
blue cohosh (*Caulophyllum thalictroides*)
cramp bark (*Viburnum opulus*)
wild yam (*Dioscorea villosa*)

The Complete Prescription for PMS Relief

Note: Unless otherwise noted, these strategies should be followed throughout the entire month, not just when symptoms occur.

Cardiovascular exercise: 30 minutes a day, 5 days a week
Calcium: 1200 milligrams daily of calcium carbonate or calcium citrate
Vitamin D (for calcium absorption): sunlight exposure 3 to 5 minutes a day, two or three days a week, or supplements of 1000 IU daily during winter months in northern climates
Light therapy (for PMDD): frequent exposure to natural sunlight, or 30 minutes of bright white light of 10,000 lux daily
Magnesium: 300 milligrams daily
Chasteberry (for PMS-related breast pain): 30 to 40 milligrams by mouth as needed for relief of symptoms

7

Making Menopause More Comfortable

WHAT YOUR DOCTOR HASN'T TOLD YOU AND THE HEALTH-STORE CLERK DOESN'T KNOW ABOUT ALTERNATIVE MEDICINE FOR MENOPAUSAL SYMPTOMS

What Your Doctor Hasn't Told You About Alternative Medicine for Menopausal Symptoms	And What the Health-Store Clerk Doesn't Know
Conventional medicine offers a wide variety of medications for menopausal problems, aside from hormone replacement therapy (HRT).	It's unknown whether there are dangers associated with long-term use of herbal HRT alternatives.
Soy products may help reduce some of the symptoms of menopause.	Whether soy should be taken as part of a diet or as a supplement—and how long your soy regimen should last
In the laboratory, wild Mexican yam looks similar to the female hormone progesterone.	Whether this extract can be successfully converted to progesterone in the human body

(continued)

What Your Doctor Hasn't Told You About Alternative Medicine for Menopausal Symptoms	And What the Health-Store Clerk Doesn't Know
Paced respiration is one of the most effective and safest techniques for relieving hot flashes.	Why more expensive treatments aren't any better
You'll find much more information about these therapies—as well as many others—in the rest of this chapter.	

Menopause, which usually occurs between the ages of 45 and 55, is not in itself a disease, although many health-care professionals treat it that way. It's a series of physiological changes that marks the end of a woman's fertility. The ovaries stop releasing eggs, and the production of female hormones undergoes a steep decline. How steep? The two key female hormones, estrogen and progesterone, drop in concentration in the bloodstream by a phenomenal 99 percent. By contrast, as men get older their levels of testosterone decline slowly over the decades. In some men, they don't decrease at all.

This precipitous drop in female hormone levels can be associated with a series of uncomfortable symptoms, including hot flashes, difficulty sleeping, vaginal dryness, and mood changes. For years, most women relied on hormone replacement therapy (HRT) to treat these symptoms.

Now that HRT has been linked to an increased risk of breast and ovarian cancers, women have been left to twist in the wind. Doctors used to automatically write out a brisk and consoling prescription for menopausal symptoms, but they are now faced with a long discussion of various options, none of them entirely attractive. Squeezed by their tight schedules, some M.D.'s have simply left the playing field when it comes to talking about complicated menopausal issues.

As a result, many women are casting about on their own for relief.

According to a study conducted by the North American Menopause Society, a stunning 80 percent of women ages 45 to 60 reported using non-prescription therapies for their menopausal symptoms. You may be one of the millions of women asking yourself: is there a good replacement for hormone replacement?

A health-store clerk might tell you that herbs like black cohosh, chasteberry, and dong quai reduce symptoms "naturally" and therefore safely. But this chapter will arm you with critical information about which alternative treatments have not yet been proven safe for the kind of long-term use most women have in mind. I'll also offer you some good news, including a combination of gentle therapies that can help you weather the storms of menopause.

HOT FLASHES FOR HIM

Men whose testosterone levels drop dramatically as a result of prostate cancer treatment also experience hot flashes.

Conventional Medicine for Menopause Symptoms: More Than HRT

Until a few years ago, menopausal women as a group were less interested in alternative treatments for their symptoms. That's because millions of them relied on HRT, a combination of estrogen and progestin. This treatment helped untold numbers of women feel like themselves again by alleviating problems like hot flashes, insomnia, and bone loss.

All that changed with the results of the Women's Health Initiative (WHI) study, which demonstrated that women who take HRT may be at increased risk for heart disease, stroke, breast cancer, and pulmonary embolism. Further studies showed that HRT increases ovarian cancer, gallbladder disease, and blood clots.

Against this bleak scenario, there remains some hope for HRT. For one, the WHI and other studies tested just one combination of estrogen and progestin—and it was a fairly high dose at that. A more recent WHI study of women using estrogen therapy alone (performed on women who did not need progestin, as they had previously undergone hysterectomies and had no need for progestin's preventive effects on uterine cancer) showed no increased risk of heart disease or stroke. It's possible that HRT taken at lower levels or in different combinations will yield fewer of these nasty side effects. Also lost in the media haze around HRT is the news that its ill effects may be reversible if the medication is taken for a short time only. There are also very early indications that estrogen might help prevent colon cancer and cataracts. Until we have more information, though, it's worthwhile to examine alternatives to HRT.

Currently, there is only one reasonable use for HRT during menopause: the temporary relief of menopausal symptoms that cannot be controlled by any other means. If you suffer from hot flashes, mood swings, or other problems so intense that you no longer feel in control of your life, try the first-line methods suggested on these pages. If these gentle treatments don't bring you relief, you might talk to your doctor about taking HRT at a low dose for a limited period of time. You can also try a short-term course of one of the herbal alternatives to HRT. These are discussed later in the chapter.

Conventional medicine offers its own form of alternatives to HRT. One of its most promising frontiers goes by the acronym SERM, which stands for selective estrogen receptor modulators. Cells possess two forms of estrogen receptors: alpha receptors and beta receptors. Alpha receptors are associated with the deleterious effects of estrogen, such as breast and uterine cancers. Beta receptors are associated with estrogen's benefits, including the protection of bone mass. The beauty of SERMs is that they bind only to those beneficial betas, producing bone protection without the cancer risk. It's also possible—although still unproven—that some SERMs can reduce the risk of heart attacks. The most popular SERM for treatment of menopausal problems is raloxifene (Evista). This drug poses its own risks, however, including a higher chance of blood clots. And it doesn't reduce symptoms like hot flashes or insomnia at all.

It's beyond the scope of this book to discuss osteoporosis in detail, but loss of bone mass is a serious concern for postmenopausal women. In addition to SERMs, most doctors recommend training with weights two or three times a week to build bone density. Consult with a qualified trainer or physicial therapist to learn the moves that are right for you.

If you're looking to cool down your hot flashes, some conventional medications other than HRT appear to help, though none is as effective. Low doses of antidepressants—including venlafaxine (Effexor), fluoxetine (Prozac), and paroxetine (Paxil)—have a decent success rate when it comes to reducing hot flashes. Blood-pressure drugs such as clonidine (Catapres) and methyldopa (Aldomet and Amodopa), also taken in lower-than-usual-doses, may offer relief. Before you take an untested alternative substance, you should ask your doctor about these tried-and-true medications.

For vaginal dryness, which can make sex painful, consider prescription estrogen creams. These topical medications improve lubrication and suppleness. Better still, they don't carry the risks of oral HRT.

As you consider the conventional options for menopause symptoms, keep this in mind: if your doctor won't make time to discuss these medications with you, it's time to find a new doctor.

The Discriminating Consumer's Guide to Menopause Alternatives

Your doctor may not have a whole lot to offer for some of the most annoying symptoms of menopause. Women who suffer from hot flashes or sleepless nights are frequently left to their own devices.

Sadly, there are people willing to take advantage of women's desperate need to relieve their symptoms. I'm especially frustrated by the multitude

THREE SIMPLE STEPS FOR RELIEVING HOT FLASHES

There are some practical ways to relieve hot flashes, one of the most frustrating symptoms of menopause. Before you turn to medications or herbs for help, give some of these at-home treatments a try:

1. *Keep it cool.* According to the North American Menopause Society, a cool environment can reduce the number of hot flashes you experience. And it's probably not surprising that warm surroundings crank up the heat of your symptoms. Some commonsense measures for staying comfortably cool include using fans, air-conditioning, or open windows. Cold drinks and food can also help lower body temperature. Try to avoid or reduce your consumption of hot or spicy food and drinks. Dress lightly whenever possible; if you must wear heavy clothing, plan ahead and wear layers that can easily be removed.

2. *Don't smoke.* Did you know that smoking cigarettes substantially increases your risk of hot flashes? And that with each cigarette you smoke, you raise the odds that your hot flashes will be more severe? So if you do smoke, quit. Now. (It's interesting to note that alcohol consumption is *not* related to the number or severity of hot flashes.)

3. *Get moving.* Roll out the yoga mat, crack open a can of tennis balls, or put on your boogie shoes, because studies indicate that daily exercise cuts your chances of having hot flashes. Be careful if you're really out of shape, however: exercise in poorly conditioned women can have the opposite effect. If it's been a while since you worked up a good sweat, check with your doctor to create an appropriate exercise regimen that lets you gradually build up your fitness level.

of claims for herbs that supposedly act as "natural HRT." This kind of overstatement could lead women to take products that, yes, might work, but might also be just as dangerous as HRT, especially in the long term.

But you don't need to shun alternatives just because some salespeople are improperly motivated by the bottom line or well-intentioned wishful thinking. There are products and therapies that have either been proven effective or hold promise for menopausal symptoms, especially hot flashes. If you know the facts, you'll know which alternatives are smart to try—and what kinds of cautions to take when using them.

You'll see that most alternatives for menopause focus on hot flashes, but you will also find some information below about menopause products that may help with sleeplessness, mood changes, and bone loss. For a more thorough discussion of disorders whose risk increases with menopause—such as heart disease, depression and anxiety, and insomnia—you can also consult the relevant chapters in this book.

ALL IN YOUR HEAD?

Over and over, studies show that placebos have a strong effect on one of menopause's most annoying symptoms: hot flashes. This doesn't mean that hot flashes are all in your head! They are a very real physiological response to a drop in hormone levels. The success of placebos in clinical trials points to a profoundly optimistic possibility: that you may be able to use your mind—not drugs or expensive alternative treatments—to control hot flashes.

You can start by trying two mind-body therapies that have already been proven to reduce hot flashes. These are paced respiration and the relaxation response, both of which are explained in this chapter. I hope that we'll soon see studies of other mind-body therapies, including hypnosis and guided imagery, for hot flashes. When so many other therapies for hot flashes contain known or potential dangers, it's simply inappropriate for the scientific community to ignore the safe therapies that might really work.

HIGHLY RECOMMENDED ALTERNATIVE TREATMENTS
FOR MENOPAUSE SYMPTOMS

Paced Respiration

Here's some welcome news if you suffer from hot flashes: in three clinical trials, a mind-body technique called paced respiration cut in half the number of hot flashes experienced by postmenopausal women. The women also reported fewer symptoms of depression and anxiety. (In these studies, paced respiration was compared with biofeedback, reading, or no activity at all.)

Now for a short course in paced respiration: get comfortable and remove all distractions. Then breathe in slowly and deeply, as if to drink air down into the very bottom of your lungs. Now breathe out, just as slowly. If you're performing this technique correctly, you should be able to feel your abdomen—not just your chest—moving in and out as you breathe.

And that's all. No money and only the most minimal time and effort. Women report the best effects when they use paced respiration at the onset of a hot flash. How long do you keep up this deep, focused breathing? Perhaps for just a couple of minutes—and perhaps longer. You may need to experiment to find the right amount of time for you.

Relaxation Response

Placebos are known to have a strong effect on hot flashes. This led scientists at the Mind/Body Medical Institute at the New England Deaconess Hospital (a major teaching hospital of Harvard Medical School) to wonder whether the mind's power could be directly harnessed to relieve this symptom. They were specifically interested in the relaxation response, a deeply relaxed, meditative state that may improve several measures of health.

These scientists worked with 33 women who were experiencing at least five hot flashes each day. These women were randomly assigned to a relaxation response group, a reading group, or a control group that simply charted their symptoms. The relaxation-response group was instructed in the technique and asked to perform it for 20 minutes every day. The reading group read leisure material for the same amount of time. None of the groups reported fewer hot flashes, but the relaxation-response group—and *only* the relaxation-response group—found that their symptoms were much less intense. Along with paced respiration, the relaxation response is one of the few menopausal alternatives that I can recommend without reservation. For more information about the relaxation response, see "How to Elicit the Relaxation Response" on pages 19 and 20.

RECOMMENDED ALTERNATIVE TREATMENTS
FOR MENOPAUSE SYMPTOMS

Phytoestrogens (Soy and Red Clover)

Soy milk at Starbucks. Edamame in the supermarket's freezer section. And rows and rows of soy and clover pills lining the shelves at the health store. A woman can hardly turn 40 these days before she's admonished to make these products part of her daily routine. That's because soy and red clover products are high in phytoestrogens, plant-based compounds that bear a chemical resemblance to estrogen.

You've probably heard some experts say that phytoestrogens produce the desirable effects of estrogen without the cancerous effects on the breast and uterus. Phytoestrogens are promoted to reduce hot flashes and improve sleep—and also ward off the heart disease, memory failure, and bone loss that so often plague menopausal women. Can you believe these claims? If so, which form of phytoestrogens—food or supplement— is most likely to help you?

The intense interest in phytoestrogens comes to us via Asia, where as few as 15 to 20 percent of postmenopausal women report hot flashes.

Compare that with the numbers in the United States, where hot flashes affect a hefty 75 to 80 percent of women, and you can see why scientists turned east in their quest for a substance to soothe this symptom.

One possible answer sits atop the kitchen tables of Asian households. Soy—which is present in products such as soy flour, soy milk, and tofu—is consumed in much larger quantities in Asia than in the West. Soy is also packed with isoflavone compounds that are one of the most potent forms of phytoestrogen. The obvious association led to the use of soy for the treatment of menopausal symptoms. Legumes and red clover, which are also excellent sources of phytoestrogens, are popular as well.

But the answer to the big question—do phytoestrogens really work?—remains elusive. Below is a look at several menopause symptoms and the evidence for phytoestrogens.

THE FLAP OVER FLAXSEED

Plenty of menopausal women are counseled to eat flaxseeds or use flaxseed oil to counteract the effects of estrogen loss. Although flaxseeds contain phytoestrogens, they do not boast the same level of estrogenic activity as the phytoestrogens found in soy, red clover, and legumes. Flaxseeds are a fabulous source of flavonoid antioxidants, however, so you can continue to enjoy them atop salads or in yogurt, or to use their oil as a dressing. Just know that they may not have as much power to halt your hot flashes as advertised.

HOT FLASHES. Most studies show that about 20 to 40 percent of the women taking a placebo have a reduction in symptoms, whereas about 30 to 50 percent of those taking soy or soy-derived supplements experience an improvement. With numbers this close, it's difficult to measure the true benefits of soy and to separate them from the placebo effect. In one promising study published in the *American Journal of Epidemiology,* women whose diets contained the most soy products or soy supplements reported the fewest hot flashes.

Red clover, a dried flower long used by Native Americans for its medicinal properties, has also been investigated for its effect on hot flashes. Although Native Americans did not use this herb for relief of menopause symptoms, red clover is now attracting notice for its high content of isoflavone phytoestrogens. As with soy extracts, there's a large placebo effect. But there's reason to be cautiously optimistic.

Most studies of red clover extract have focused on its supposed ability to reduce hot flashes. In two well-conducted trials, red clover was no more effective than a placebo. In two *other* trials, however, red clover shot past placebo in its ability to control hot flashes. One of these studies used a smart strategy for gauging the placebo effect. In this study, 30 Dutch women received a placebo for four weeks and saw their hot flashes decline by an average of 16 percent. Then the women were given either red clover or placebo for an additional twelve weeks. Remarkably, the red-clover group saw their hot flashes decline by 44 percent—but there was no significant change in the placebo group. To help support these findings, we need to conduct larger studies on red clover and hot flashes.

HEART DISEASE. At home I have a box of oatmeal-soy cereal that proclaims, "Diets low in saturated fat and cholesterol that include 25 grams of soy protein may reduce the risk of heart disease." This statement was approved in 1999 by the Food and Drug Administration. Soy has indeed been found to lower heart-disease risk by reducing cholesterol. But if you don't like soy in your cereal—or if your palate rejects tofu, soy burgers, soy milk, and other soy products—don't expect to get the same cardiovascular results from popping a pill. It's far from clear whether isolated soy isoflavones (that's a fancy name for soy supplements) have a cholesterol-lowering effect. Nor do we know whether other forms of phytoestrogens, including red-clover supplements, can improve your cholesterol profile.

There is also preliminary evidence that dietary soy (not supplements) and red-clover extracts can increase the flexibility of arterial walls, thereby cutting your risk of high blood pressure and eventual heart disease. Before you rely on either product to avert heart disease, however, wait for further studies—and make sure you practice the proven heart-healthy strategies discussed in the chapter 10, "Preventing Heart Disease and Stroke."

MEMORY LOSS. Both animal and clinical studies indicate a relationship between estrogen and cognitive functions such as memory. The memory center of the brain, known as the hippocampus, is rich in estrogen receptors, and brain scans of women receiving estrogen show increased blood flow in this site. So it stands to reason that phytoestrogens might have a similar effect. Here's what the science shows so far:

In a small study published in *Psychopharmacology,* college students who were on diets rich in soy showed improved memory when compared with those eating a low-soy diet. And in a randomized, controlled clinical trial at the University of California, San Diego, 56 postmenopausal women who were not taking estrogen were given either soy isoflavone or an identical-looking pill. After six months, the women were asked to perform a series of cognitive tests. On every single test, the soy isoflavone group put in a consistently better performance. In some tests their showing was nearly 20 percent stronger when compared with the placebo group. This study shows real promise, but further evidence is needed before I can recommend soy supplements for memory loss.

BONE LOSS. Now that HRT is no longer a long-term option for maintaining bone strength, many women have been turning to isoflavones as a way to stave off the prospect of osteoporosis. But it's too early to depend on isoflavones for bone health.

In a pattern that will look familiar to you by now, there are some studies that seem to show that isoflavones from soy and red clover increase bone mineral density. In one of these studies, women taking high levels of soy isoflavones showed a small but statistically significant increase in the density of the lumbar spine, a region where osteoporosis can strike hard. But another study of soy isoflavones failed to produce any improvement in bone density. Research is needed to compare dietary soy and soy supplements with weight training, which is known to increase bone mass, and the conventional medications listed earlier in this chapter.

BREAST CANCER. Breast-cancer rates are much lower in Japan than in the West, so the Japanese diet has also been the locus of interest in breast-cancer research. The Japan Public Health Center–Based Prospective Study on Cancer and Cardiovascular Diseases Group looked at soy consumption specifically. In this study of more than 21,000 Japanese women age 40 to 59, those who consumed the most soy in their diet had the lowest risk of developing breast cancer. But in a sobering twist, there are lab studies indicating that soy supplements may actually *stimulate* breast cancer cell growth. Obviously, we need much more information about the relationship between breast cancer and phytoestrogens before even considering them for long-term use. For now, phytoestrogen supplements shouldn't be used at all by women with a high risk of breast cancer. These women should also go lightly on their consumption of dietary soy.

Given the shaky state of knowledge about soy and the absence of long-term studies, my recommendation is to approach soy isoflavone supplements with the same kind of caution you'd use with HRT. That is, take soy isoflavone supplements only if you experience severe menopausal symptoms—and then use them for no more than six months. Certainly, no women with a family history of breast cancer or other risk factors should take phytoestrogen supplements of any kind until it's clear whether they cause breast cancer or prevent it.

DOSAGE AND SIDE EFFECTS: The existing clinical studies on soy isoflavones have experimented with a range of doses, from 30 milligrams a day to 104 milligrams. It appears that as little as 30 milligrams may yield some benefits. I usually encourage people to take the lowest doses possible;

the different commercial preparations probably vary in their actual strength, however, because the dosage given on a product's label isn't always accurate. So if you do wish to try a short-term course of isoflavone supplements, I'd recommend taking between 60 or 70 milligrams. Since the best effect occurs when the dose is divided, try spreading those 60 or 70 milligrams into two or three doses throughout the day. For women without a family history of breast cancer, there appear to be few downsides to dietary soy or soy isoflavones—though you might develop an allergy to soy and soy products. If you want the best results, you'll need to pack in as many soy servings per day as you can stand.

Red-clover supplements come with another set of warnings. One form of clover contains a potent anticoagulant, which can interfere with blood clotting. These supplements may make it difficult for you to stop bleeding if you're cut or experience other traumas, brain hemorrhages, or stomach ulcers. Red clover also lacks the track record of soy foods, because unlike soy, which has been on dinner plates for millennia, red clover has never been part of the human diet. And it's never been used on a long-term basis for hot flashes.

I recommend taking red clover only for hot flashes that truly interfere with your quality of life and that cannot be brought down to an acceptable level with more conservative measures, such as changes in lifestyle or paced respiration.

PHYTO POWER

It remains unclear whether soy supplements (pills) work for menopausal complaints, and the possible side effects of taking soy supplements for long periods of time have not yet been adequately investigated. But it may make sense to increase your intake of *dietary* soy—that is, food products made from soybeans. Below are several food sources of phytoestro-

(continued)

gens. Although the isoflavones in soy most closely mimic the structure and function of estrogen, it can make sense to add several of these products to your diet. Even if some of them—such as flaxseeds, which I discuss on page 136—have not been proven to have effects on menopause symptoms, they have several other health benefits that make them smart dietary choices.

Note: Women with a family history of breast cancer should soft-pedal their consumption of soy, as there is a possible link between breast cancer and soy intake.

alfalfa and clover sprouts
fruits (especially apples)
green tea
legumes (including chickpeas, split peas, pinto beans, and lima beans)
lentils
seeds (including flaxseeds)
sesame
soy (including tofu, tempeh, soy flour, and soy milk)

If you decide to try red clover, I suggest a product called Promensil, which is the preparation used most often in clinical studies. Take a tablet two times each day for no more than six months.

Black Cohosh (Cimicifuga racemosa)

Black cohosh is a popular alternative remedy for menopausal complaints. In fact, this herb enjoyed a distinguished history of use long before the term *alternative medicine* became part of contemporary vocabulary. Native Americans felt that black cohosh root relieved menopausal symptoms such as hot flashes, mood changes, and sleep problems; in the early 1900s, it was a main ingredient in patent medicines for "female complaints." Today, a black-cohosh preparation is approved in Germany for menopausal as well as menstrual problems.

Did our ancestors know something about black cohosh that we don't? Many women, frustrated by the side effects of HRT, are willing to take the gamble: in 1999 alone, sales of black cohosh reached $34 million, according to the *Nutrition Business Journal.* They are probably much higher today.

If you talk to a black-cohosh enthusiast, you'll probably hear about dozens of studies in the 1980s and 1990s that supposedly proved the effectiveness of black cohosh at reducing hot flashes. But these studies didn't do a very good job at using placebos to measure the real effects of the herb. Nor were the studies blind, meaning that the investigators might have unconsciously affected the outcome. And none examined the long-term effects, positive or negative, of black cohosh.

Lately, there have been far more rigorous and dependable clinical trials. These have produced mixed results. One study in Germany found that black cohosh did not prove to be significantly better than the placebo in reducing hot flashes. But it was at least equal to estrogen— and *much* better than the placebo—at reducing other complaints, including sleep disturbances and mood problems. As in so many other studies discussed in this chapter, the large placebo effect for hot flashes makes it difficult to present any definitive proclamations about the efficacy of black cohosh. Nevertheless, there is enough precedent for the use of black cohosh that I'm willing to recommend it—but only for short-term relief of severe symptoms that don't respond to gentler therapies such as paced respiration.

DOSAGE AND SIDE EFFECTS: I suggest a product called Remifemin, which contains a standardized amount of black cohosh. Take it in doses of 40 to 80 milligrams twice daily. You may need to take black cohosh for one to three months before you notice an effect—and you should not take it for more than six months, as its long-term effects are unknown. Never take black cohosh as a lifelong replacement for HRT.

Be careful not to confuse black cohosh with its blue cousin (called blue cohosh, of course). Some products used by herbalists or midwives for childbirth include both black cohosh and blue cohosh, so steer clear of these. This should be not a problem if you use Remifemin exclusively. Do not take any form of black cohosh if you have hypertension or heart problems, as this herb can dilate blood vessels and add to the effect of any antihypertensive medications you are taking. It also shouldn't be used if there's any possibility you're pregnant. That's not a consideration for most menopausal women, but remember that until your periods have stopped for twelve months you may still be capable of conceiving.

Other than the warnings above, there are a few mild side effects that are possible with black cohosh use, including upset stomach, headaches, dizziness, breast pain, and weight gain.

BEWARE THIS HOT-FLASH TRIGGER

The herbal remedy yohimbe, which has gained popularity as a supposed aphrodisiac, can bring on hot flashes as well as other and more severe side effects. Avoid this product.

ACCEPTABLE ALTERNATIVE TREATMENTS
FOR MENOPAUSE SYMPTOMS

Acupuncture

Here's an interesting study that points to a powerful mind/menopause connection: in a Swedish study, menopausal women were randomly divided into two groups. The first group was given electroacupuncture, a variation on traditional acupuncture in which mild electrical stimulation is applied to the needles. The other women received a kind of sham acupuncture in which needles are inserted at the usual points but not at the depth thought to produce acupuncture's effects. The fascinating result? *Both* groups reported a significant reduction in their hot flashes. There was no real difference between the two groups. (The study's investigators also looked at whether acupuncture improved sleep for these women, but they found no effect.)

This leads me to conclude that it wasn't acupuncture itself that worked its magic on hot flashes. Perhaps it was the soothing, quiet time spent in the treatments; perhaps it was the human interaction between patient and acupuncturist; or perhaps it was the subjects' hope that acupuncture could help. Whatever the reason, there is powerful evidence here that hot flashes can be altered by mental states.

If you want to try electroacupuncture for your hot flashes, be my guest. (Regular acupuncture has not been well tested for its effects on this symptom.) It's safe (as long as your practitioner is using disposable needles), and many people find it deeply relaxing. If you don't mind spending the money on a series of treatments, you might find relief from this uncomfortable symptom. I suggest using the same frequency and duration of treatments used in the Swedish study: twice weekly for two weeks and then once weekly for six additional weeks.

Chasteberry (Vitex agnus-castus)

Chasteberry, a fruit of the chaste tree, has been used for women's health problems since Hippocrates was drafting his famous medical oath back in ancient Greece. In contemporary times, chasteberry is sold as a treatment for hot flashes. However, there are no good studies showing that chasteberry is effective for menopausal symptoms.

DOSAGE AND SIDE EFFECTS: Despite the lack of proof, chasteberry appears to be safe if you want to try it. Use it only when other and better-researched therapies have failed, and then take it just for a short time, as there are no long-term studies of chasteberry's effects. Anyone taking medications that affect dopamine levels, such as l-dopa, should avoid chasteberry. Those of you who are in the early stages of menopause and taking oral contraceptives should be aware that chasteberry can interfere with the Pill's effectiveness. Other side efects include fatigue, headaches, gastrointestinal upset, rash, and hair loss. If you are prepared to encounter these potential problems, you can try 40 milligrams of chasteberry daily, either in capsules or in an aqueous-alcoholic solution.

Evening Primrose (Oenothera biennis)

Does the yellow primrose, a North American wildflower, hold the literal seeds of promise when it comes to relief from hot flashes? Some people believe that because an extract of yellow primrose seeds, called evening primrose oil, is high in the omega-3 oils that do so much good elsewhere in the body, it can reduce hot-flash symptoms. But they appear to be wrong. In a study published in the *British Medical Journal,* 56 women were randomly divided into two groups. The first group received four 500-milligram capsules of evening primrose oil daily; the other got a placebo that was in a similar liquid form. After twenty-four weeks, the two groups showed little difference in the number of hot flashes experienced.

If you have severe hot flashes that don't respond well to other treatments, it's safe for you to give evening primrose oil a try, though I'm dubious of its effectiveness.

DOSAGE AND SIDE EFFECTS: Try 2 or 3 grams of evening primrose oil daily, dividing this amount into two or three smaller doses over the course of the day. The side effects of this herb are mild and include nausea and diarrhea.

Wild Mexican Yam (Dioscorea villosa)

Advertisements for wild Mexican yam enthusiastically refer to this extract as "natural progesterone" and claim that it reduces hot flashes, mood changes, depression, and insomnia. There's a half-truth behind this pronouncement. Wild yam does indeed contain diosgenin, an ingredient that is similar to progesterone, one of the hormones whose levels plunge during menopause. You can imagine the train of thought: if wild yam resembles one of the hormones menopausal women lack, then perhaps it can restore the hormonal balance and reduce symptoms. But it just doesn't work that way.

Although wild yam may chemically resemble progesterone, it does not convert into progesterone where it counts—in the human body. An excellent clinical study shows that wild yam is no better than a placebo when it comes to reducing hot flashes.

DOSAGE: There is no real justification for using wild Mexican yam, but it appears to be safe to try, at least for short durations. If you'd like to determine for yourself whether it turns down the heat of hot flashes, try an Australian product called BioGest, which contains wild Mexican yam extract along with vitamin E. Apply it twice daily to the buttocks, arms, legs, and abdomen.

Homeopathy

There have been no convincing studies that compare homeopathic treatments against placebo when it comes to menopause symptoms. Although I'm wary of homeopathy—the substances are so diluted that it's difficult to imagine how they could possibly work—many menopausal women claim to obtain relief from a variety of symptoms with these products. That kind of anecdotal evidence isn't nearly as good as clinical trials, but homoeopathic products are so safe and so cheap that there's not much downside to giving them a try.

Remedies that are often recommended for menopause include *Amyl nitrosum, Lachesis mutur, Nux vomica, Natrum muriaticum, Belladonna, Cactus grandiflorus, Caulophyllum, Gelsemium, Ignatia amara, Murex, Pulsatilla, Sulfur, Ustilago, Maydis, Zincum valerianum,* and *Sepia.* Passionate advocates of homeopathy often say that the best effects are achieved only by consulting with a homeopath, but this significantly increases the price of this highly controversial therapy.

DO NOT USE THESE ALTERNATIVE TREATMENTS
FOR MENOPUASE SYMPTOMS

Chiropractic Manipulation

Some chiropractic practitioners have proposed that menopausal problems are related to small dislocations, called subluxations, in the spine. These subluxations can supposedly be treated with—surprise—a series of visits to your local chiropractor for spinal adjustments. But there's no evidence to back this theory up, and the most reputable chiropractors stay away from claims that their services can improve much other than pain along the spine.

Ginseng (Panax ginseng)

The term *ginseng* is derived from *panacea,* meaning "cure-all." And if you've witnessed the way this herb is promoted for menopause symptoms, you might believe it indeed cures all: it's supposed to reduce hot flashes, stress, memory loss, and depression. Yet the scientific literature is surprisingly bare when it comes to ginseng and menopause. The best study, reported in *Menopause: The Journal of the North American Menopause Society,* suggests that ginseng has no effects on hot flashes or other

GINSENG . . . OR NOTHING?

One reason to be wary of ginseng, aside from its lack of evidence for menopause symptoms, is the dubious quality of the products for sale. In one study, only 25 percent of commercial "ginseng" preparations were found to contain any ginseng at all. And several products contained large amounts of caffeine. It makes you wonder whether the sense of well-being reported by some ginseng users could have been more easily obtained with a jolt of java.

menopausal symptoms, though it appears to improve the subjects' over-all sense of well-being.

I encourage my colleagues to conduct some tightly controlled studies on ginseng, as there's just not enough evidence to help women make good decisions about this highly popular herb. Until we know about ginseng, I do not recommend its use for menopausal symptoms. Under no circumstances should it be used if you're taking prescription anticoagulants, as it increases the risk of bleeding. Ginseng should also never be taken with monoamine oxidase inhibitors such as phenelzine (Nardil), tranylcypromine (Parnate), and isocarboxazid (Marplan), because it interferes with the metabolism of these drugs.

Dong Quai (Angelica sinensis)

For more than a thousand years, practitioners of traditional Chinese medicine have used dong quai in combination with other herbs to relieve menopausal complaints. Here in the West, dong quai is more commonly taken by itself. There have been several clinical studies on dong quai, and none of them has shown a real reduction in menopausal symptoms. Some people will tell you that dong quai's long history means that it's safe to use anyway when nothing else works. Don't believe them. This herb contains an essential oil that's carcinogenic. That's not good for anyone, especially menopausal women, who are at a newly increased risk for breast cancer. Dong quai can also cause excessive bleeding and shouldn't be taken by women on anticoagulants.

It's possible, however, that dong quai works differently when used in traditional Chinese medicine, where it's prescribed as part of an individualized combination of herbs. Perhaps some of the other herbs mitigate its dangers or work in synergy with dong quai to produce a more powerful benefit. But that possibility has never been studied properly. Like much else in traditional Chinese medicine, it must remain a fascinating mystery for now.

Kava Kava (Piper methysticum)

Kava kava is often promoted as a treatment for the psychological symptoms that can occur in menopause. At least two reasonably good studies have been conducted indicating that kava kava can reduce anxiety and depression in postmenopausal women. Before you reach for the kava bottle, however, know this: this herb has been known to cause liver failure. Whatever comfort kava kava offers, it's not worth the risk. If you'd like to learn more about kava kava, see chapter 5, "Taming Depression and Anxiety."

Licorice (Glycyrrhiza glabra)

Licorice root forms the basis for several Chinese menopause remedies. But neither those herbal combinations nor licorice alone has been adequately investigated in clinical studies. Besides, licorice has some alarming side effects: hormonal problems, heart disease, and high blood pressure. Licorice should never be taken with diuretics, as both substances reduce potassium; together, they could lead to severe potassium depletion and serious heart problems. Fortunately, people who love licorice candy will be happy to know that it's not made from the real—and dangerous—thing.

The Complete Prescription for Menopause Symptom Relief

GENERAL MEASURES

Keep cool.

Cardiovascular exercise: 30 minutes daily, at least 5 days a week

Weight training: two or three times weekly

Paced respiration: perform as needed at the onset of a hot flash.

Relaxation response: 20 minutes daily

Soy products (only for women without a family history of breast cancer): add as many servings to your diet as you can tolerate.

ADDITIONAL PHARMACEUTICALS FOR SPECIFIC PROBLEMS

Note: These drugs will be prescribed depending on the results of clinical evaluation.

Estrogen cream (for vaginal dryness): as prescribed
Fosamax (alendronate sodium) (for bone loss): as prescribed
Evista (raloxifene hydrochloride) (for bone loss): as prescribed
Miacalcin (calcitonin-salmon) (for bone loss): as prescribed
Antidepressants (for hot flashes and mood changes): as prescribed
Catapres (clonidine) (for hot flashes): as prescribed

FOR FURTHER RELIEF
Take only one of these therapies at a time and use for no more than
   six months unless otherwise noted.
Black cohosh (Remifemin): 40 to 80 milligrams taken twice daily
Soy isoflavone extracts: 60 to 70 milligrams, divided into two or
   three doses throughout the day
Red-clover extract (Promensil): two tablets or pills daily
Hormone-replacement therapy: at a prescribed low dose (for no
   more than five years)

8

Revving Up
Male Libido

What Your Doctor Hasn't Told You About Alternative Medicine for Men's Libido Problems	And What the Health-Store Clerk Doesn't Know
Prescription medications for flagging libido are very expensive and come with side effects.	Which of the herbal alternatives are safe—and which may kill you
Ginseng may be an effective alternative and costs only 6 cents per dose.	How much to take and for how long
A decline in blood levels of DHEA is associated with impotence in men under 60.	Whether DHEA supplements can kick an aging sex drive into high gear
	(continued)

What Your Doctor Hasn't Told You About Alternative Medicine for Men's Libido Problems	And What the Health-Store Clerk Doesn't Know
L-arginine may work in a manner similar to Viagra to improve sexual functioning.	The results real men have experienced in clinical studies of this supplement.
You'll find much more information about these therapies—as well as many others—in the rest of this chapter.	

With aging there is a normal decline in male sexual function. Testosterone, the male sex hormone, decreases—and with it goes some of a man's muscle mass, bone strength, and, of course, libido. As a man grows older, it may take longer to become aroused. Erections are usually less firm and ejaculations less forceful, and the time between erections lasts longer. Conservative estimates suggest that at least 30 million men experience difficulty maintaining an erection. Yet these difficulties do not need to interfere with healthy and enjoyable sex.

The success of Viagra and newer drugs in helping men maintain erections has led to numerous alternative therapies that also claim to improve libido and erectile function. Since Viagra costs more than $8 per dose, many men consider responding to the ubiquitous e-mail advertisements for potency herbals and aphrodisiacs. Some turn to physicians who offer testosterone injections. In this chapter, I'll describe these alternative therapies and answer the important questions: Do they work as well as Viagra? And do they have fewer side effects?

More Solutions Than Just Viagra

In 1998, Viagra was introduced, and men discovered that diminished sexual function was no longer something they just had to live with. Although Viagra doesn't rev up sexual desire, it *does* help the body to maintain erections when taken anytime between 30 minutes and four hours before it's needed. Now, as you undoubtedly know from the barrage of television and print advertising, there are newer prescription medications that have challenged Viagra. These drugs, Levitra and Cialis, last longer than Viagra. Cialis can be effective for up to three days.

The side effects of Viagra, Levitra, and Cialis are similar and include headache, flushing, and runny nose. There may also be a subtle change of vision, causing objects to appear blue. This is the source of many jokes about these drugs, but in a small percentage of the population this effect can develop into a serious eye problem. Occasionally, these drugs can also cause priapism, a condition in which an erection lasts for four or more hours. Again, this is a side effect that many people laugh about, but it's a painful, even dangerous condition that must be treated immediately.

Viagra, Levitra, and Cialis also interact with prescription drugs, including nitrates (nitroglycerin), taken for heart disease, and alpha-blockers (Cardura, Minipress, and Hytrin), which are used to lower blood pressure. And of course, with a cost of several dollars per dose, another of these drugs' side effects is damage to your bank account. With so many perils surrounding conventional drugs, many men would prefer a safer, lower-cost alternative.

To Crank Up Your Libido, Bring Down Your Weight

It was once thought that erectile and arousal problems were purely psychological in origin. These days, we tend to assume that libido woes are a matter of biochemical imbalance, to be cured with a pill. But did you know that you can improve sexual performance without drugs or psychotherapy?

Recent studies strongly suggest that exercise and appropriate weight loss are effective bedroom boosters. According to the Health Professionals

Follow-Up Study, regular physical activity appears to reduce impotence risk by nearly a third. So does weight maintenance. In the same study, men who were substantially overweight were 30 percent more likely to experience impotence than their fit-and-trim counterparts. When obese men lose weight, many of them regain their sexual functioning.

The Discriminating Consumer's Guide to Male Libido and Impotence Alternatives

As you might suspect, there are plenty of folks looking to make a quick buck off a man's search for increased libido and improved erectile function. Are there any legitimate remedies available? Let's look at the offerings.

ACCEPTABLE ALTERNATIVE TREATMENTS FOR MEN'S SEXUAL PROBLEMS

Ginseng (Panax ginseng)
Like Viagra, ginseng relaxes the muscles in the penis and allows it to fill with blood. In one study of 90 men with erectile dysfunction, nearly two-thirds experienced improvement in their symptoms when using this herb. As a point of comparison, only 30 percent of men given a placebo reported better sexual performance. This trial is only preliminary—it was fairly small and took place in Korea and Brazil, where strong scientific standards are not always in place—but it's promising. Two other small trials have yielded good early results for red ginseng as well.

Ginseng has a few more checks in the "plus" column. Although it hasn't been subjected to long-term studies, it appears relatively safe when taken for short periods of time. Its cost—about 6 cents per dose—is ginseng's other great advantage. So why not try this herb before paying through the nose for Viagra, Cialis, or Levitra?

DOSAGE AND SIDE EFFECTS: Take 1 gram of ginseng three times daily. (Unlike Viagra, which is taken as needed, ginseng must be taken on a continual basis.) The safety of long-term use hasn't been tested.

Ginseng increases the risk of bleeding, so do not take it if you're using prescription anticoagulants. Ginseng also interferes with the metabolism of certain drugs, including monoamine oxidase inhibitors such as phenelzine sulfate (Nardil), tranylcypromine sulfate (Parnate), and isocarboxazid (Marplan).

L-arginine

Viagra works by enhancing the action of nitric oxide as it relaxes the muscles in the blood vessel walls in the penis and therefore helps maintain erections. L-arginine, an amino acid that increases blood levels of nitric oxide, has also been marketed to enhance sexual performance.

There have been only three small pilot studies on L-arginine for erectile dysfunction. One showed no effect, but the other two demonstrated a significant improvement. There is some evidence that men with low levels of nitric oxide respond well to L-arginine, but that those with normal levels do not see an effect with this supplement.

It's too early to say for sure whether L-arginine works; some men may reasonably feel it's worth a try before paying the big bucks for a conventional drug. Be aware, however, that unlike Viagra, which is taken only as needed, you'll need to ingest daily doses of L-arginine and keep taking them if you want any effect to continue. Amino acids can be powerful substances, and their effects when taken as supplements are not well understood. Do you really want to put such large quantities of as untested product into your body?

DOSAGE AND SIDE EFFECTS: If you want to try L-arginine, you can take 3 to 5 grams per day. In the small, short-term studies conducted so far, the main side effect of L-arginine has been a small but significant drop in blood pressure, so exercise caution and consult your physician while using this product.

DO NOT TAKE THESE ALTERNATIVE TREATMENTS FOR MEN'S SEXUAL PROBLEMS

Androstenedione

The rumored use of androstenedione by several major-league baseball players has powered sales of this hormone. Profits from "andro" have sailed out of the ballpark as men hope their purchase will pump up their strength, virility, and bedroom prowess. But aside from the popular belief that andro is partially responsible for powerhouse plays on the ballfield, there's no evidence that androstenedione does much of anything for anyone. Hormones are notorious substances that can have unpredictable effects on the human body, especially when used for long periods of time. With so little evidence, there's just no good reason to take this one.

DHEA (dehydroepiandrosterone)

DHEA is a steroid that the body converts into male and female sex hormones. This fact, along with our knowledge that DHEA levels take a nosedive at about the same time sexual functioning starts to decline, has led to excited speculation that DHEA can replenish long-gone libido. But the evidence for DHEA remains weak at best.

When the Massachusetts Male Aging Study followed veterans over a period of many years, they found that of the seventeen hormones and steroids they measured, a decline of DHEA was most strongly associated with erectile dysfunction in men under age 60. This preliminary finding spurred further research, none of which has yielded the kind of smash-bang results everyone was hoping for. In one of the more positive studies, 40 men were randomly assigned to receive either DHEA or a placebo.

Those who got the DHEA reported an improvement—but only a slight one—in their potency problems when compared with those who took the placebo. I don't find these results convincing enough to recommend DHEA. These weak results, along with DHEA's potential side effects—including an increased risk of breast or prostate cancer, unwanted hair growth, acne, and male breast enlargement—earn this supplement a place on my "Do Not Use" list.

Ginkgo Biloba

Ginkgo biloba is most often used to enhance mental functioning, and some people believe that it's also an all-round tonic that can take libido up a notch as well. But there is simply no evidence suggesting that ginkgo biloba improves sexual functioning. You're better off trying exercise or losing some weight.

Testosterone

Hormonally speaking, men have it easy. Whereas women suffer the effects of a 99 percent decline in estrogen levels during menopause, men experience a slower and far less dramatic drop-off in testosterone. In some lucky men, testosterone declines only by subtle amounts. Nevertheless, many have asked the question: Since slowly sinking levels of testosterone result in decreased libido, why not just give aging men a new supply of this hormone?

For some men, the answer is clear: sign me up! And it's true that testosterone works. Not only does it increase sex drive, it can strengthen your muscles and bones while helping you shed excess flab. But before you roll up your sleeve for a costly testosterone injection (taking this hormone as a pill doesn't get it into the bloodstream, so you'll need either a shot or a skin patch), know this: testosterone stimulates the growth of prostate cancer cells, increases LDL cholesterol (the bad kind), and decreases HDL cholesterol (the good kind). Furthermore, there are no long-term studies of testosterone replacement, so any decision to receive this hormone must be taken with caution. I recommend waiting a few years, as a number of drug companies are working on medications called SARMs (selective androgen receptor modulators) that could have the beneficial effects of testosterone without the negative effects on your prostate and heart. There are also a few long-term studies of testosterone replacement therapy supported by the government that should be finished in upcoming years.

Yohimbe (Pausinystalia yohimbe)

Yohimbe is sold with great fanfare via e-mail solicitations and in health stores. When I went to a local health food store and asked for recommendations for decreased libido, the clerk showed me a bottle of yohimbe and said with great enthusiasm and emphasis that it was guaranteed to "improve things." I could see why this herb is such a best seller. But yohimbe presents a classic case of "buyer beware."

Yohimbe is a chemical isolated from the bark of an evergreen tree that grows in the jungles of western Africa. It is sold as an aid for impotence and erectile dysfunction, but the evidence for yohimbe is extremely poor.

What makes yohimbe most alarming is the severity of its side effects. The FDA has received reports of kidney failure, seizures, and even death. If that's not enough to warn you away, yohimbe can also exacerbate kidney or liver disease, angina, heart disease, and high blood pressure, as well as psychological and neurological problems. Anyone who takes yohimbe—and again, I strongly recommend that you don't, given that ginseng offers a much safer alternative—should avoid eating food containing tyramine and caffeine. That means no coffee, tea, chocolate, liver, cheese, or red wine, among other foods. It's obvious why yohimbe isn't a best-seller in France!

The Complete Prescription for Revving Up Male Libido

Cardiovascular exercise: 30 minutes daily, at least 5 days a week

Weight loss: if you are seriously overweight

Ginseng: before taking prescription medications for sexual problems, consider trying ginseng first. Although it lacks strong evidence, ginseng appears safe for short-term use, and it's much less expensive than prescription drugs. 1 gram taken three times daily.

Prescription medications, such as Viagra, Cialis, Levitra: as prescribed

9

Improving
Prostate Health

WHAT YOUR DOCTOR HASN'T TOLD YOU AND THE HEALTH-STORE CLERK DOESN'T KNOW ABOUT ALTERNATIVE MEDICINE FOR ENLARGED PROSTATE	
What Your Doctor Hasn't Told You About Alternative Medicine for Enlarged Prostate	And What the Health-Store Clerk Doesn't Know
Saw palmetto has demonstrated the same effectiveness as conventional prostate drugs, with fewer side effects.	Why you must *always* tell your doctor if you're taking saw palmetto
Certain plant-based foods may reduce your risk of enlarged prostate.	There's no evidence that supplements derived from these foods have a similar effect.
Pygeum africanum, beta-sitosterols, and bee pollen are all marketed as prostate-health supplements.	Which ones are worth your time— and which lack a track record of safety
You'll find much more about these therapies in the rest of this chapter. For information about alternative medicine for prostate cancer, see chapter 12, "Cancer Prevention and Treatment."	

Almost half of older men have symptoms related to an enlarged prostate. The prostate is a chestnut-shaped organ that sits below the bladder and surrounds the urethra, the tube that conducts urine away from the bladder and out of the body. As the prostate grows larger, it squeezes the urethra and produces changes in the pattern of urination. These can include less forceful urination, leakage, and—most bothersome—the need to get up many times at night to visit the bathroom. Although an enlarged prostate doesn't increase the risk of prostate cancer in and of itself, a large prostate can make it difficult for your doctor to spot a tumor. Prescription medications are expensive and often accompanied by serious side effects. Surgical removal of the prostate, although usually very successful, is an even more drastic option that most men would prefer to avoid if possible.

That's why so many of us are intrigued by evidence that Egyptian physicians four millennia ago used plant extracts to treat prostate problems. Today, some Europeans are taking a page from this ancient culture: in Germany, 90 percent of men with enlarged prostates are treated with phytochemicals (chemical compounds found in plants). This chapter will discuss a number of these phytochemicals, including one that is as effective as prescription medications in reducing mild to moderate prostate symptoms with fewer side effects. For men with enlarged prostates, this supplement offers a less expensive and more tolerable alternative to conventional drugs. By relieving the intensely irritating symptoms of an enlarged prostate, it may also help avoid the need for surgery.

Conventional Prostate Treatments: Are They Really Your Best Bet?

There are two main classes of conventional drugs that slow prostate growth. Alpha reductase inhibitors such as finasteride (Proscar) inhibit the conversion of testosterone into dihydrotestosterone (DHT), the hormone that directly stimulates prostate growth. Alpha adrenergic receptor blockers, which include tamsulosin hydrochloride (Flomax) and terazosin hydrochloride (Hytrin), work by relaxing the prostate and bladder muscle. Both classes of drugs have serious side effects, such as dizziness and problems with ejaculation. Their high cost is another drawback, especially for folks with no or limited insurance coverage for prescription medications.

Should the prostate start causing serious troubles, such as obstructing urine from leaving your body, it's time to remove the prostate surgically. Sometimes men find lesser symptoms, such as nighttime urination, so disruptive that they also opt for surgery. Surgical removal of the prostate is one of the most common operations in the United States, with 100,000 performed each year. As I mentioned before, prostate surgery comes with a high success rate—but there also can be significant complications, such as impotence and urinary incontinence. If annoying symptoms are your main complaint, it's important to find a less radical treatment, whether conventional or alternative, that is both effective and affordable for you.

The Discriminating Consumer's Guide to Prostate Alternatives

When conventional medications for prostate health don't work or when they bring unpleasant side effects (including damage to your bank account), there's an array of alternatives available. You won't need to spend lots of time deciding among them, however, because one supplement stands out as the safest and most effective. There are also some dietary measures that may protect you from prostate enlargement.

HIGHLY RECOMMENDED ALTERNATIVE TREATMENTS
FOR PROSTATE ENLARGEMENT

Saw Palmetto (Serenoa repens)

Saw palmetto is produced from the berry of the saw palm tree, which you might see if you live in or visit the southeastern United States. Native Americans used saw palmetto to treat both infertility and prostate inflammation, and early in the twentieth century it made an appearance on the list of official drugs in the U.S. Pharmacopeia.

The Native Americans were right, at least partially: saw palmetto works for prostate inflammation. A number of clinical trials have shown that men who take saw palmetto are twice as likely to experience improvement of prostate symptoms than those who receive a placebo. How does saw palmetto stack up against conventional medications? Dead even, for mild to moderate prostate problems. It produces the same amount of relief as its more expensive prescription counterparts.

Saw palmetto appears to be a natural alpha-reductase inhibitor without the vicious side effects of the conventional drugs. This phytochemical may perform double duty as an agent against inflammation and testosterone. There is no evidence that saw palmetto stops prostatic enlargement, but it does increase urinary flow and limit those late-night trips to the bathroom. Although there are no long-term studies of saw palmetto's safety, this phytochemical has a historical track record of use with few serious problems. Just as significant, saw palmetto costs somewhere between $6 and $20 per month, compared with about $65 for the prescription drug finasteride (Proscar).

DOSAGE AND SIDE EFFECTS: Take 160 milligrams of saw palmetto extract twice daily with meals. Make sure the product you buy is standardized to 90 percent lipsterolic content. I prefer Permixon, a commercial preparation that has been used most often in clinical trials. Avoid

---

WARNING: SAW PALMETTO CAN HIDE SIGNS
OF PROSTATE CANCER

Saw palmetto can be an effective treatment for the symptoms of prostatic enlargement. Never try to diagnose yourself with this disorder, however. Any man with urinary problems needs to be checked out by a doctor, who will rule out other—and possibly more serious—underlying causes. Be especially sure to tell your health-care practitioner if you are taking saw palmetto, which may impede proper diagnosis by altering your symptoms. Saw palmetto may also throw off the results of diagnostic tests for prostate cancer.

---

saw palmetto teas, as they may not contain saw palmetto's active component.

Because saw palmetto and prescription medications for prostate enlargement appear to have the same mode of action, avoid taking both of these products at the same time. You should know that gastrointestinal bleeding and headaches have been reported with saw palmetto use.

RECOMMENDED ALTERNATIVE TREATMENTS
FOR PROSTATE ENLARGEMENT

Isoflavones

Did you know that lentil soup may lower your risk of enlarged prostate? Beans, tofu, and soy milk could have a similar effect. Each of these foods is high in isoflavones, which are plant-based compounds that have estrogen-like effects. The evidence isn't conclusive yet, but there is a strong argument for adding isoflavones to your diet. One study of Mormon men who drank soy milk showed a reduced risk of prostate enlargement, and men in Hong Kong, where soy products are popular, tend to have lower rates of enlarged prostate than Western men.

Beware of shortcuts. There's no evidence that isoflavones have a similar protective effect when isolated from the other compounds in foods and packaged as supplements. (You'll often see these items sold as red-clover or soy supplements.) Instead, ladle up a heaping bowl of split pea soup, dig into a bean burrito, or toast your health with a soy-milk latte every day.

Pygeum (Pygeum africanum)

Pygeum africanum (also known as simply "Pygeum") is an extract produced from the bark of an African prune tree and has been used in Europe since 1969 for relief of mild to moderate prostate symptoms. How this extract might work against prostatic enlargement is not yet fully understood, but studies on animals (not humans) have shown an anti-inflammatory effect.

The human studies on *Pygeum africanum* are preliminary but promising. In 12 out of 13 small clinical trials, *Pygeum africanum* produced improvements in symptoms such as urine flow, amount of urine left behind in the bladder, and the need to urinate at night. The patients who took *Pygeum africanum* reported about the same number of side effects as the men taking a placebo; most of these side effects were gastrointestinal and included problems such as nausea, diarrhea, or constipation.

So why don't I recommend this product wholeheartedly? Many of the studies did not fully disclose the statistical methods used to determine their results, and none used a standardized scale of symptoms to measure the supplement's effects. Nor did any compare *Pygeum africanum* against conventional prostate medications. If other products, including saw palmetto, haven't worked for you, it may nevertheless be reasonable to try *Pygeum africanum*. Be aware that although it caused few side effects in clinical studies, no one has tested this product over the long term.

DOSAGE: Take 50 to 100 milligrams of *Pygeum africanum* daily.

ACCEPTABLE ALTERNATIVE TREATMENTS
FOR PROSTATE ENLARGEMENT

Beta-Sitosterol

Beta-sitosterol is an extract usually derived from South African star grass, although it can also be produced from other plants. Beta-sitosterol contains phytosterols, which—in theory—can bring down inflammation and reduce prostate complains. Early studies indicate that beta-sitosterol improves urinary flow and other symptoms, but most of these trials did not meet high scientific standards. Many of them used beta-sitosterol products that did not contain consistent amounts of the active ingredient. I'm also concerned that these trials were too small to truly gauge the effects of this phytochemical.

Side effects of beta-sitosterol appear to be minor and infrequent; about one percent of men who take the remedy complain of gastrointestinal problems. In addition, there are no good long-term studies of beta-sitosterol. That's also true for saw palmetto and *Pygeum africanum,* but at least those products have a centuries-long history of use. I'm waiting for better studies of beta-sitosterol, and so should you.

DO NOT USE THESE ALTERNATIVE TREATMENTS
FOR PROSTATE ENLARGEMENT

Pollen Extracts (Cernilton)

European men often rely on pollen extracts to relieve the symptoms of an enlarged prostate. The commercial preparation Cernilton is especially popular. If you inquire about this product at the health store, you may hear about a study showing that 75 percent of men who use Cernilton experience a reduction in urinary urgency and frequency—but be wary. Although placebos are known to have a strong effect on urinary frequency, this trial failed to test Cernilton against a group using a placebo. Unfortunately, no placebo-controlled studies of Cernilton or other pollen extracts have yet been performed.

Until the evidence is stronger, I suggest you avoid pollen extracts. Many people develop allergic responses to pollen, a risk not worth taking when saw palmetto appears to work so well.

The Complete Prescription for Relief of Prostate Symptoms

Saw palmetto (for mild to moderate symptoms): 160 milligrams of a product standardized to 90 percent liposterolic content, taken twice daily with meals

Conventional medications: as prescribed, but not together with saw palmetto

Surgery: for severe symptoms when more conservative approaches have failed

Isoflavone-rich diet: eat plenty of beans, soy products, and lentils (but don't use isoflavone supplements).

10

Preventing Heart Disease and Stroke

WHAT YOUR DOCTOR HASN'T TOLD YOU AND THE HEALTH-STORE CLERK DOESN'T KNOW ABOUT ALTERNATIVE MEDICINE FOR PREVENTING HEART ATTACK AND STROKE

What Your Doctor Hasn't Told You About Alternative Medicine for Preventing Heart Attack and Stroke	And What the Health-Store Clerk Doesn't Know
Fish oils can lower blood pressure and improve the function of your arteries.	Which fish oils are most effective
Red yeast rice extract has several cholesterol-lowering compounds, one identical to a common prescription medication.	The reasons you should not yet replace your current cholesterol-lowering drug with this supplement
Folic acid is one of the keys to heart health.	How much folic acid you should take
Hawthorn may help the heart function more efficiently.	Why you should take this herb only under supervision of your doctor

(continued)

What Your Doctor Hasn't Told You About Alternative Medicine for Preventing Heart Attack and Stroke	And What the Health-Store Clerk Doesn't Know
The Japanese government has approved coenzyme Q_{10} for the treatment of congestive heart failure.	The reasons this supplement is not yet recommended for use in the United States and elsewhere
Adopting the Mediterranean and More Diet can be the best way to reduce your risk of having a heart attack.	Which foods form the basis of this enjoyable dietary program
You'll find much more information about these therapies—and many others—in the rest of this chapter.	

Keeping up with the latest news about vascular health has become America's newest spectator sport. As if in a game of championship tennis, contrasting opinions volley back and forth. If you've followed the debate on fish consumption, you know just what I mean. First, headlines trumpeted the good news: fatty fish can protect your arteries and heart. Then some experts challenged this advice, explaining that many types of fish contain dangerous levels of mercury. Farmed fish was recommended instead. *Then* we learned that farmed fish have other contaminants. Now fish-oil supplements look like the best way to protect your heart. But even fish oils have their problems.

This scenario plays itself out with all kinds of advice about how to keep your arteries clear. The back-and-forth game continues until we, the spectators, nod off in exhaustion and confusion.

Except that vascular health isn't really a game. Most of us will die from diseases that are caused by the closure of key arteries that supply blood to the heart and brain. If you want to fight off heart attacks, strokes, and related killers, you need to understand the latest and best information about conventional and alternative treatments that claim to keep your arteries clear.

This chapter is meant to put *you* in control by clearly stating your best options for warding off heart disease and stroke. After reading it, you won't feel so bewildered in the drugstore or health store, because you'll have narrowed down your shopping list to the supplements that actually work. (You won't even have to *look* at the others on the shelves.) This chapter also contains my Mediterranean and More Diet, which incorporates the best and latest dietary information into a simple and pleasurable eating plan. When you're done reading, you can reward yourself by taking time out to enjoy one of the many relaxation therapies that appear to clear your arteries and block disease.

You and Your Arteries

Arteries (tubes that carry blood away from your heart and to the rest of your body) begin life as flexible structures with walls so smooth and clean they could pass the cardiac version of the white-glove test. But when something disturbs the lining of your blood vessels, arterial plaque can result. This plaque restricts the blood vessel's flexibility and narrows its inner channel, making it more difficult for blood to pass through. The condition is called arteriosclerosis (hardening of the blood vessels) and may eventually cause the blood vessel to spasm or close. When heart and brain blood vessels go into spasm, angina (chest pains brought on by exertion) and "little strokes," called transient ischemic attacks, occur. When the arteries close, the consequences are heart attacks and strokes.

Two of the most important factors in preventing and treating arteriosclerosis are maintaining a healthy balance between your good cholesterol (HDL) and bad cholesterol (LDL) and keeping your blood pressure under control. While doctors have known for decades that elevated blood cholesterol and high blood pressure are major risk factors for heart disease and stroke, we have unearthed some surprising facts about how to keep both of them check. This new information affects the medications you take, what you can put on your breakfast plate, and what you should buy in the supplement aisles.

Conventional Medications to Prevent Heart Disease and Stroke

The current emphasis in medical offices is to treat high blood pressure, elevated cholesterol, and impaired sugar metabolism aggressively, in hopes of preventing heart attacks and strokes. Doctors know that it's best to accomplish these goals through lifestyle changes, including exercise, good nutrition, and weight management. But if these strategies fail, it's time for prescription drugs. There are many drug classes available, including the following:

- Cholesterol-lowering statins (Zocor, Lipitor, Mevacor, Crestor, Pravachol)
- Blood pressure medications: diuretics (Lasix, Hygroton, Naturetin, Edecrin, Bumex, hydrochlorothiazide), calcium channel blockers (Norvasc, Procardia, Cardizem, Veramil), beta blockers (Tenormin, Lopressor, Coreg, Inderal), angiotensin-converting enzyme (ACE) inhibitors (Lotensin, Vasotec, Altace, Monopril, Zestril), and angiotensin receptor blocker antagonists (Cozaar, Diovan)
- Blood-sugar-lowering medications (Precose, Actos, Avandia, Glucotrol, Micronase, Glucophage, and various insulin medications)
- Blood-thinning medications, including enteric-coated baby aspirin

Each of these classes of medications comes with side effects that can range from mild to intolerable. These include muscle pains, dizziness, drowsiness, depression, dehydration, hearing loss, anemia, skin rashes, asthma, nausea, fatigue, loss of libido, liver problems, and gastrointestinal problems. But even with their long list of potential problems, there is much positive evidence for these drugs. When high blood pressure, high blood sugar, and high cholesterol don't respond to lifestyle changes, a doctor who doesn't recommend drugs is practicing medicine at a level below the standard of care. If you don't take advantage of their benefits, you could open the door to heart disease, kidney disease, stroke, or blindness. Should you take one of these drugs and suffer severe side effects, have a frank discussion with your doctor—and be prepared to experiment with several drugs until you and your doctor hit on a combination that's right for you. Unlike other classes of drugs, these medications sometimes work best if you take low doses of several brands rather than a high dose of just one. (This doesn't mean it's okay to combine alternative heart-health supplements with conventional medications without telling your doctor first. The results could be unpleasant or even dangerous.)

If you already have heart disease or have suffered from a stroke—or if you suffer from risk factors such as high cholesterol—alternative medicine isn't much of an alternative to the excellent medications available.

Medicine and lifestyle changes can keep you off these drugs in the first place, however. Around 90 percent of heart disease can be avoided through diet, exercise, and weight control, and perhaps by taking some well-chosen supplements or employing mind-body treatments. Similar strategies can prevent most cases of stroke. If you're one of the unlucky millions who have already experienced a heart attack or stroke, some of these alternatives can play an adjunct role in fending off a repeat occurrence. If not, let some smart alternatives keep you out of the cardiologist's office in the first place.

The Mediterranean and More Diet

When I visit Rome, I'm always amazed at how many old Italian men I see walking the boulevards. According to conventional medical wisdom, most of these guys should have died long ago! They are often smoking, and plenty are overweight. The most vigorous exercise I see them perform is a game of bocci. Yet their life expectancy is about the same as ours. Their secret? The Mediterranean diet.

Actually, the term *Mediterranean diet* is a bit misleading, since there is no single diet followed by every Mediterranean citizen. Thanks to the vibrantly individual cultures—Spanish, Greek, Italian, Moroccan, French—that make their home alongside this sunny sea, there's a wide culinary diversity in the region. These folks do have a few things in common, however: a love of bright flavors, avoidance of fast food and its trans-saturated fats, some serious consumption of olive oil, and an impressively low rate of heart disease. Extract the shared elements of their diets—fish, nuts, legumes, whole grains, fruits, vegetables, olive oil, tomato products, wine—and you have a tasty recipe for keeping your arteries clean.

The foods in question all contain at least one of several substances thought to keep your arteries in fighting trim. One class of these substances is the antioxidants, which appear to prevent plaque buildup on artery walls. Fiber, which can lower bad cholesterol by up to 20 percent in people with elevated cholesterol levels, is also present in most of these Mediterranean staples. Nuts and olive oil contain monounsaturated fats that improve your cholesterol profile. Fish brings the bonus of the heart-protective omega-3 fatty acids.

I recommend some minor adjustments to the Mediterranean diet, mostly based on strong evidence for including additional foods. That's why I call it the "Mediterranean and More" approach to eating. Each food in my Mediterranean and More Diet, below, is backed by science and my sworn testimony to their deliciousness.

The Mediterranean and More Diet:

- *Enjoy fruits and vegetables, whole grains, legumes, garlic, nuts, and tomato sauces.* Each of these classical elements of the Mediterranean diet is rich in at least one substance (most frequently fiber, antioxidants, or good fats) that keeps your ticker ticking and your blood flowing freely to your brain. Berries are one of the best sources of antioxidants, so tuck into a bowl of strawberries, blueberries, raspberries, or other berries every day.
- *Make olive oil your choice for cooking.* Olive oil is the principal source of dietary fat in the Mediterranean region and contains flavonoids as well as the good fats that can improve your cholesterol profile. Don't turn up the flame too high; extreme heat destroys the beneficial monounsaturated fats.
- *Get adequate amounts of omega-3 fatty acids.* The low rates of cardiovascular disease among Mediterranean cultures are directly related to their heavy reliance on fish for protein. Fish—particularly fatty fish such as tuna, salmon, mackerel, and herring—is rich in omega-3 fatty acids. These fish oils go to work on many aspects of heart disease: they lower blood pressure, improve the function of artery walls, and decrease blood clotting. The Mediterranean and More Diet does *not* recommend you eat more than two servings of fish per week, however, because of the possibility of mercury contamination. (Fatty fish are especially likely to contain mercury.) You can also get your omega-3s from fish-oil supplements, which are discussed later in the chapter.
- *Toast your health once or twice a day.* Although red wine is the most famous component of the traditional Mediterranean diet, any kind of alcoholic drink—whether it's chardonnay or a cosmopolitan—appears to be good for your blood vessels when used in moderation. Alcohol raises the good cholesterol and

removes the bad kind from your bloodstream. It's possible that alcohol also prevents blood clots from forming, thus keeping your blood circulating normally. Make sure that you drink in moderation: indulge in more than two drinks daily and you'll increase your chances of certain forms of heart disease, liver disease, and stroke. Women should limit themselves to one drink a day; more than that and they may be in greater jeopardy of developing breast cancer.

- *Introduce soy products into your diet.* Soy is not a traditional Mediterranean food, but there's good reason to include it here. Both the federal government and the American Heart Association recommend consumption of 25 grams of soy protein daily. Studies show that people who eat this admittedly high amount of soy experience a significant decrease in bad cholesterol levels—around 13 percent. Triglycerides (a type of fat linked to increased risk of heart disease) also drop by about 10 percent. It can be tough to make room on your plate for so much soy (depending on your choices, you may need between two and four servings of soy products to get the recommended 25 grams), but it may be worth adding this ingredient whenever you can. Don't, however, force yourself to eat steamed cakes of tofu if you dislike its bland flavor or texture. Instead, try pan-searing tofu and serving it in a curry sauce for a crispy main course. You can toss out the tofu altogether and enjoy the sweetness of soy milk in your whole-grain breakfast cereal. Or pop edamame (boiled green soybeans) straight from the bag. They are much tastier than you might think and make a satisfyingly crunchy snack. I keep a sack of edamame in the freezer and thaw a few to munch on each day.

- *Enjoy a chocolaty conclusion to your meals.* Mediterranean cultures aren't known for their love of sweets, so dark chocolate definitely puts the "more" into my Mediterranean and More

Diet. Like many of the other foods found in this diet, chocolate contains flavonoids, powerful antioxidants that may prevent bad cholesterol from oxidizing into the arterial plaque that can cause heart attacks. Recent studies also indicate that chocolate can relax arteries. The more cocoa in your chocolate, the more antioxidants you'll get, so go for the dark or bittersweet varieties. They have more cocoa and less fat than milk chocolate.

- *Go easy on meat, saturated fats, and fatty dairy products.* Mediterraneans minimize these foods, which are known to raise your risk of arteriosclerosis. How about replacing your afternoon latte and cookie with a favorite Mediterranean snack: figs stuffed with walnuts?
- *Drink green or black tea.* Both drinks contain antioxidants. There's been so much confusion surrounding tea that I've given this pick-me-up its own entry later in the chapter.

A LITTLE DINNER WITH YOUR OLIVE OIL?

Of all Mediterranean countries, the island of Crete boasts the highest consumption of olive oil: about 20 gallons per person every year! They also enjoy the lowest rate of heart disease in Europe and are three times less likely to develop heart disease than their U.S. counterparts.

Fitness

When it comes to preventing heart disease and stroke, the very best medicine is exercise. Even small amounts of exercise can bring these big payoffs to your cardiovascular system:

- Lowering bad (LDL) cholesterol
- Raising good (HDL) cholesterol

- Improving aerobic fitness
- Reducing blood pressure
- Reducing triglyceride levels
- Improving the body's metabolism of sugar

Don't have time to exercise? Let's look at evidence from two very busy groups of people: doctors and women (married women are the least likely of us to find time for exercise). The 1999 Health Professionals Study at Harvard shows that male physicians who made time for just one vigorous workout per week reduced their risk of stroke by 21 percent. According to the Nurses' Health Study, women who tallied up just 1 to 2.9 hours of brisk walking each week saw their risk of heart disease plummet by nearly a third. If you exercise more frequently, your risk of both diseases drops even further.

Studies of longevity show that exercise produces only modest increases in life span. But exercise produces an enormous difference in the quality of your time here on Earth. Your risk of disability is reduced and your chance of leading a productive, vital life skyrockets if you can work in weekly exercise sessions. To increase the likelihood that you'll stick with a fitness regimen, choose a workout you enjoy. For example, I get bored quickly on exercise machines. Fortunately, I live in Southern California and can get out to play tennis and golf two or three times a week. I also try to avoid elevators and walk as much as possible. For those of you in less pleasant climes, put your television in front of your workout equipment and watch your favorite show while you improve your cardiovascular fitness.

The Discriminating Consumer's Guide to Alternatives for the Treatment and Prevention of Heart Disease and Stroke

For all our scientific advancements, there remains much that we don't know about keeping arteries clean. For that reason, a number of supplements and other alternative treatments for heart and stroke prevention are highly popular. Step into your health store and you may be shocked by the number of options. Should you take hawthorn? Vitamin E? Use red yeast rice extract to lower your cholesterol? You might be tempted to give up and just go relax somewhere—but with proponents of meditation, biofeedback, and cognitive-behavioral therapy all claiming that these treatments decrease your risk of heart disease and stroke, just which method of relaxation will you choose?

Don't worry. I've done the legwork for you. In this section, I've winnowed that exhaustive (and exhausting) list of options down to the few that actually work. Now you really *can* relax!

HIGHLY RECOMMENDED ALTERNTATIVE TREATMENTS FOR HEART DISEASE AND STROKE PREVENTION

Fish oils (omega-3 fatty acids)

Fish oils are the alt-med superheroes against heart disease. They protect you from the villainous duo of high blood pressure and blood clots that can cause heart attacks. (They can even fight depression and boost brain function, but that's for other chapters.) Heart-attack patients who add fish or fish-oil supplements to their diets reduce their risk of death from a subsequent heart attack by as much as 57 percent.

Although I usually recommend getting nutrients from food, supplements of fish oil can be a smart choice. That's because dietary sources of fish oils—including fatty fish such as wild tuna and salmon—can be contaminated with mercury. Farm-fed fish have other contaminants, such as dioxins and PCBs.

DOSAGE AND SIDE EFFECTS: There are several fish-oil products on the market. Find one that contains both EPA (eicosapentaenoic acid) and DHA (docosahexanoic acid) and take 1 gram per day. Larger doses, of 10 to 15 grams, are used as a treatment for elevated triglycerides, which are fats that put you at risk for heart disease and stroke. These large doses also cause intestinal side effects that most people find seriously uncomfortable, however.

Normal doses of fish oils can lead to side effects that include a fishy smell on the breath, gastrointestinal upset, and increased bleeding. Some people experience more pronounced side effects than others. About a month after I started fish-oil supplements, I began to experience abdominal cramps and diarrhea. After an extensive and inconclusive medical workup, I diagnosed myself with fish-oil intolerance. I stopped the supplements, and my GI problems disappeared. To get my fish-oil hit, I try to make it to my favorite sushi bar at least once a week. (Fatty fish—including mackerel, herring, salmon, and tuna—are best.)

Folic Acid and Vitamin B₁₂

Homocysteine doesn't receive as much press as cholesterol or blood pressure, but when it comes to your heart, high homocysteine levels are bad news. People whose homocysteine levels are in the top 10 percent of the population are twice as likely as the rest of us to develop heart disease or suffer a stroke. (If you don't know your homocysteine level, ask your doctor to perform a test.) Luckily, there's an easy way to reduce homocysteine: by getting adequate amounts of folic acid and vitamin B_{12}.

If you take a daily multivitamin or generally follow a good diet, you may still not be getting enough folic acid and vitamin B_{12}. To keep homocysteine under control, you need between 650 and 1000 milligrams of folic acid every day. Because folic acid isn't absorbed well by the body, it's difficult to get those amounts from your diet. And multivitamins tend to supply you only with the recommended daily allowance of folic acid (the synthetic version of folate), which is a mere 400 milligrams. To be sure that you're keeping homocysteine under firm control, you'll need to take a folic acid supplement in addition to eating good food sources of this nutrient. These include fortified grain products, black-eyed peas, lentils, and cooked spinach.

Vitamin B_{12} also helps lower homocysteine. But as you get older, your stomach begins to produce less acid. That sounds like a good thing, but the less acidic environment encourages the growth of digestive bacteria that just love to eat vitamin B_{12}. It's estimated that 10 to 25 percent of older Americans don't get enough vitamin B_{12}. If you're over 55, you should take vitamin B_{12} supplements in addition to folic acid. (Vitamin B_6 also lowers homocysteine levels, but can produce serious side effects, as discussed on page 123. Folic acid and B_{12} will do the trick for you.)

DOSAGE: Get 800 micrograms of folic acid from food and supplements daily. If you're 55 or older, also take a daily dose of 1 milligram (1000 micrograms) of vitamin B_{12}.

Mind-Body Therapies

Did you know that being down in the dumps can be hard on your heart? Numerous studies have shown that depression is associated with a higher risk of heart disease. Other psychosocial factors—including anxiety, hostility, a bad work environment, and low social support—also make it more likely that you'll end up in the hospital's cardiac ward. These findings have naturally led to the hypothesis that if stressful mental states can contribute to heart disease, perhaps calmer ones can produce the opposite effect. Can biofeedback and other mind-body treatments really bring down the risk of heart problems?

The answer is yes. According to an article published in the *Archives of Internal Medicine,* heart-attack patients who participated in mind-body treatments such as relaxation or classes to reduce angry, stressed-out "type A" behavior were almost 50 percent less likely to die or experience repeat heart attacks than those who did not use these therapies. The patients who practiced mind-body therapies also showed greater reductions in risk factors such as blood pressure, heart rate, and cholesterol levels.

In another study, 153 patients who'd experienced cardiac arrest were divided into two groups and followed for two years. One group underwent mind-body therapies consisting of relaxation, biofeedback, cognitive-behavioral therapy, and lessons in coping with depression, anger, and anxiety. The second group took health-education courses about the importance of eating a low-fat diet and engaging in physical activity. After two years, there were seven deaths in the health-education group but only one in the group that received mind-body therapies.

With this kind of success rate and practically no side effects (aside from a calmer, happier life), mind-body treatments are a great way to prevent heart attacks. Choose the therapy that most appeals to you and go for it!

Another mind-body therapy, meditation, has less evidence behind it and is discussed separately in this chapter.

RECOMMENDED ALTERNATIVE TREATMENTS FOR HEART DISEASE AND STROKE PREVENTION

Green Tea

After water, tea is the world's favorite beverage. When a number of population studies linked green and black tea consumption with protection from heart disease, it seemed we all had another reason to pour a cup. One well-controlled clinical trial, conducted by scientists at Vanderbilt Medical Center and performed in Shanghai, examined the effects of tea extract versus a placebo on 240 Chinese men, all with mildly elevated cholesterol levels. After twelve weeks, those who had received the green tea extract had a 16 percent reduction in LDL cholesterol. Nutrition science bolstered tea's heart-healthy reputation further by demonstrating that both black and green tea are rich sources of catechins, which are powerful antioxidants.

Not all research on tea is positive, however. A study of 17,000 older Harvard and University of Pennsylvania alumni showed that tea drinkers developed cardiovascular disease in the same numbers as those who preferred other beverages. There was only a small and insignificant decrease in the risk of stroke for the long-term tea drinkers. But the subjects in this study drank primarily black tea. This stands in contrast to the Chinese study, which used green tea extract.

Although I usually recommend green tea because of its higher antioxidant content, there's no reason to convert from black tea if you really love it. It appears to provide some antioxidant protection, although slightly less than that of green tea. Since both green and black tea taste so good, I suggest people avoid the pills and enjoy a nice cup of the real thing.

If you're a confirmed coffee drinker (and if your heart is not sensitive to caffeine), there's good news for you as well: the alumni study discussed above also showed no relationship between coffee ingestion and subsequent risk of heart disease. Moderation in excess can be deadly—or at least deadly dull—so as long as the caffeine isn't keeping you awake at night, drink as much coffee as you like. Java is one of life's healthier vices.

Meditation

In 1975, Harvard doctor Herbert Benson made headlines (and the best-seller list) with his announcement that meditation and what he called the "relaxation response" could lower blood pressure. (Note that the relaxation response involves a special meditative technique and is different from relaxation as discussed earlier in the entry on mind-body

WHAT GINGKO IS GOOD FOR:
PERIPHERAL VASCULAR DISEASE

The harmful effects of fatty deposits aren't limited to those arteries leading to your heart and brain. When plaque accumulates in blood vessels that supply other parts of your body, especially the legs and feet, you can develop a condition known as peripheral vascular disease. The main symptom of this condition is a cramping sensation in the legs when you're walking around. Although peripheral vascular disease isn't a direct cause of heart attack and stroke, it is associated with a higher risk of these problems.

So it's good news that gingko, one of the oldest herbal medicines around, can ease the symptoms of peripheral vascular disease. Several studies have shown that when compared with a placebo, gingko increases the distance that people with this disorder can comfortably walk. It may not be a cure for peripheral vascular disease, but anything that helps you get moving is definitely a good thing. Butcher's broom, another popular supplement for peripheral vascular disease, shows some promise but has not yet been proven to work.

DOSAGE AND SIDE EFFECTS: Take 40 to 50 milligrams of a gingko product called EGb 761 (available from German suppliers) or an American gingko extract standardized to 24 percent gingko flavone glycosides and 6 percent terpene lactones. Gingko is a blood thinner and can increase bleeding. If you are going in for surgery and are taking gingko (or any herbal supplement), tell your doctor.

therapies.) More recently, David Eisenberg, another Harvard doctor and one of alternative medicine's brightest stars, reviewed hundreds of studies to determine whether meditation can in fact reduce blood pressure. He found that this therapy works—but only minimally, with an average drop of just 3 millimeters in systolic pressure and 1 millimeter in diastolic blood pressure. That's not nearly enough to reduce heart-disease risk in most people with high blood pressure.

There are simply not enough quality studies of meditation and its effects on hypertension to come to a conclusion. One persistent problem is that the available research has often been performed by investigators with ties to organizations that promote transcendental meditation. I hope that unbiased scientists will take a closer look at this therapy and give us some reliable answers.

Obviously, meditation should never serve as a substitute for conventional blood-pressure medications. It remains an entirely safe and thoroughly enjoyable form of relaxation, however. If you find that meditation leaves you feeling calmer and better equipped to handle life's stresses—by all means, do it as often as you can.

Magnesium

It's been proposed that low levels of magnesium are related to an increased risk of cardiovascular disease. The Harvard School of Public Health analyzed the dietary magnesium levels of 40,000 male health professionals and then followed them for ten years. Men with the highest intake of magnesium had 30 percent fewer incidents of heart disease than men with the lowest intake. The Honolulu Heart Study, published in 2003, produced strikingly similar results.

These findings are interesting on the surface, but the studies failed to take into account that certain lifestyle habits go together. In the Harvard study, men who took magnesium supplements were also more likely to be nonsmokers who exercised regularly. They also tended to get more potassium, folic acid, vitamin E (though this supplement's effectiveness against heart disease remains in question), and cereal fiber. If the intake of potassium—a mineral crucial to heart health—is factored out, the study shows no relationship between magnesium and heart disease.

No matter what the studies say, magnesium remains an important mineral for several body functions, including digestion (many antacids and laxatives contain magnesium salts as an active ingredient). Although magnesium is present in communities with hard water, it's a good idea for those of you with soft water to take magnesium supplements.

DOSAGE AND SIDE EFFECTS: Take 320 milligrams daily of elemental magnesium if you live in a soft-water area. The amount of elemental magnesium in different magnesium compounds varies enormously: 1 gram can contain from 54 to 603 milligrams, depending on whether you use magnesium gluconate, magnesium sulfate, or magnesium oxide. I recommend taking magnesium sulfate, which contains about 99 milligrams of elemental magnesium per gram. The main side effect of magnesium salts is diarrhea.

Niacin

Niacin, also called nicotinamide or nicotinic acid, is a B-complex vitamin. It's found in many multivitamins at a dosage of 14 to 16 milligrams. At this low dose, niacin has no side effects. However, many Americans have elected to use much higher doses of niacin (up to 3000 milligrams a day) to lower their cholesterol levels.

In a national study published in the *American Heart Journal* in 2000, patients with peripheral artery disease were given niacin along with several other interventions, with the goal of lowering the patients' cholesterol. Not only did niacin lower cholesterol, it also acted as an anticoagulant by lowering key clotting chemicals and thus helped in a second way to prevent heart attacks and strokes.

Niacin appears to work well, but it's important to know about its side effects. Many people develop bad headaches with niacin. Others experience intense flushing and/or feelings of warmth in their face, neck, and chest. You can alleviate this problem by using sustained-release preparations and by taking aspirin or ibuprofen 30 minutes before taking a dose of niacin. (You may also adjust to the flushing and headaches after a few weeks. Many people do.) Niacin can also cause gastrointestinal symptoms. To reduce your chances of getting this side effect, take niacin with meals. High doses of niacin can also cause peptic ulcer disease and liver damage. Niacin can increase your blood glucose levels to the diabetic range and send your blood uric acid levels to levels usually seen only in cases of gout. Rarely, it can cause muscle problems and interfere with blood clotting.

DOSAGE: If you want to take high doses of niacin to lower your LDL cholesterol, treat it as you would a prescription medicine that carries many side effects. Start taking niacin under a physician's supervision, and start with about 0.5 gram per day. If you don't experience problems, you can slowly increase the dose to 1 to 3 grams daily.

ACCEPTABLE ALTERNATIVE TREATMENTS FOR HEART DISEASE AND STROKE PREVENTION

Hawthorn

The hawthorn shrub has been a foundation of Chinese and European herbal medicine since ancient times, but only in the late 1800s did it become principally known as a heart tonic, reputedly able to improve blood circulation, lower blood pressure, prevent heart disease, and treat heart failure.

Clinical studies of hawthorn's ability to lower cholesterol and blood pressure have been inconsistent, but the high antioxidant content of its fruits, leaves, and flowers suggests that hawthorn might—at least in theory—prevent the oxidation of LDL cholesterol.

Although I don't yet recommend using hawthorn for high cholesterol, it does make the heart function more efficiently. This action is very similar to that of digitalis, a prescription medicine made from the foxglove plant. (Although scientists once speculated that hawthorn might interfere with the effects of digitalis, a 2002 study at the University of Michigan showed that this is not the case.) Several other studies show that hawthorn can reduce symptoms of heart failure—but only when hawthorn is used in conjunction with conventional medical treatment.

The side effects of hawthorn are intestinal upset, drowsiness, headache, nausea, heart palpitations, falls, dizziness, drowsiness, sedation, hypotension, and exacerbation of arrhythmia. I caution you against using hawthorn as a replacement for conventional heart medicine, as all the positive studies of hawthorn have used it as an adjunct to medical treatment. Hawthorn should never be the sole treatment for heart failure.

DOSAGE: Even though hawthorn's effects are not yet fully understood, patients with heart failure can try it under the supervision of a doctor. Unfortunately, few standardized extracts of hawthorn are available in the United States. One of them, HeartCare, is a good option. Heart-Care's recommended dosage ranges from 80 milligrams twice a day to 160 milligrams three times a day (and always take this product with meals).

Stanols and Sterols

Plants contain fats called stanols and sterols. These fats displace cholesterol in your digestive tract and can lower your blood cholesterol levels by about 10 percent. If you have high cholesterol, a 10 percent reduction may not be enough. In theory, stanols and sterols are nevertheless a wise addition to your prescription cholesterol medicine, because these plant fats can more than double the effectiveness of cholesterol-lowering statin drugs.

There's a catch, however. According a meta-analysis of clinical trials and the National Cholesterol Education Program, you need at least 2 grams a day of sterols and stanols to reduce your risk of heart disease. Although small concentrations of sterols and stanols are present in soybeans, nuts, grains, and oils, it's nearly impossible to get this recommended level from your diet. Manufacturers have responded to this dilemma by creating foods that are fortified with sterols and stanols. Most of these food products are spreads like Benecol, Take Control, and Smart Balance OmegaPlus, although fortified orange juice is also available. Additional fortified foods are probably in the pipeline.

Although I don't recommend using fortified margarine or butter products (because the fats in margarine and butter make them poor choices for anyone, especially people at risk for heart attack or stroke), the evidence for fortified orange juice is promising. In a study conducted at the University of California at Davis Medical Center, 72 people with mildly elevated cholesterol drank sterol-fortified orange juice for eight weeks. Another group received a placebo orange juice that did not contain sterols. The sterol group showed a 12 percent reduction in their LDL cholesterol levels.

I'm concerned that many fortified products give little information about the quantity of sterols or stanols they contain. As a consumer, you'll have to use your savvy and read labels to draw out as much information as possible. Because sterols and stanols may lower absorption of fat-soluble compounds such as carotenes, you'll need to make sure you eat plenty of vegetables while taking sterol- and stanol-fortified products.

The most bothersome problem is that there are no long-term studies of sterol and stanol products. It's not even clear yet which sterols and stanols have cholesterol-lowering powers. Use caution before committing to regular use of these products. I plan to wait for more information before I make them a part of my own diet.

Garlic (Allium sativum)

Garlic supplements have been shown to lower cholesterol and blood pressure, prevent blood clots, and ward off arteriosclerosis . . . *if* you're a lab rat or rabbit.

Human studies of garlic supplements, however, have been inconsistent. Some appear to show that garlic supplements have a small but significant effect on blood pressure and cholesterol, while others show no effect at all.

To be fair, it's hard to run good studies of garlic supplements. Their distinctive taste and odor make it easy for subjects to sniff out the difference between garlic and a placebo. Although deodorized garlic preparations are available, most studies have used strong-smelling dried garlic or garlic oil, putting many of those findings into question.

Garlic supplements cause unpleasant side effects, including bad breath and body odor. These side effects are minor, but with findings that are so weak, I wouldn't waste my money on garlic supplements. Instead, I enjoy the ultimate in home health care: my wife is Italian and a great chef, so we enjoy plenty of fresh garlic on our food. Not only do we enjoy our flavorful meals, we may receive a little heart protection as well.

DOSAGE: I prefer taking a fresh clove (as an ingredient of sauces or other foods) daily. If you really want to try garlic supplements, you'll need to find a garlic preparation that contains 1.3 percent allicin (read the label carefully; many products contain amounts that differ from this standard) and take 400 milligrams daily.

Coenzyme Q_{10} (Ubiquinone)

As part of the cellular machinery that converts oxygen into energy, coenzyme Q_{10} is a powerful antioxidant. It's been proposed that coenzyme Q_{10} can prevent heart disease by blocking oxidation of LDL cholesterol, and there are reports that it's beneficial in the treatment of hypertension, angina, and heart attacks.

Although your body produces coenzyme Q_{10} on its own (and also through dietary sources, especially organ meats, which unfortunately are not a healthful food choice), it's also sold as a nutrition supplement. In fact, the Japanese government has already approved coenzyme Q_{10} as a prescription drug for the treatment of congestive heart failure. The FDA, on the other hand, has approved coenzyme Q_{10} for limited use in the treatment of rare mitochondrial disorders, but *not* for heart disease or other conditions.

Although I am excited about the prospects for this supplement, there are few quality studies that have measured its effects on heart health. In one of these studies, 46 patients with severe congestive heart failure were randomized to receive either coenzyme Q_{10} or a placebo. Subsequent heart-performance studies showed no difference between the two groups. In another study, 30 Australian patients with heart failure were enrolled in a controlled study of coenzyme Q_{10}. Although blood levels of coenzyme Q_{10} doubled in those patients receiving the supplement, there was no change in their heart function.

It's difficult to balance these results against the enthusiasm of the Japanese government. I do not currently advocate taking coenzyme Q_{10}, although I'm eagerly awaiting the results of future studies that may resolve the confusion surrounding this supplement.

DOSAGE: If you plan to try coenzyme Q_{10} anyway, use a dose of 100 to 200 milligrams daily. Side effects of short-term use include diarrhea, rash, and photophobia (extreme sensitivity to light), but they are not common. There are no long-term studies of coenzyme Q_{10}, so I do not recommend using this supplement for longer than six months at a time. It's interesting to note that if coenzyme Q_{10} does prove to be beneficial in further studies, people taking statins will have to take higher doses of this supplement. That's because statins substantially reduce levels of coenzyme Q_{10}. If you try coenzyme Q_{10} and want to know whether it's having a positive effect, you might ask your doctor for a cardiac function test to gauge any improvement.

DO NOT USE THESE ALTERNATIVE TREATMENTS FOR HEART DISEASE AND STROKE PREVENTION

L-arginine

In 1998, the Nobel Prize went to researchers who discovered that nitric oxide (not nitrous oxide, which is laughing gas) performs several important biological functions. Not only is it a neurotransmitter critical for good memory and sleep, nitric oxide also relaxes the walls of your blood vessels, making them more flexible. Inflexible, stiff blood vessels contribute to high blood pressure and the development of plaque in your arteries, sending you down the road to heart attack and stroke.

What's the connection between nitric oxide and L-arginine? L-arginine is an amino acid, one of the building blocks of protein; by ingesting it, you can increase blood levels of nitric oxide. This scientific fact has led to a boom in products containing L-arginine. Some manufacturers actually labeled their products with claims that they could stop heart disease and prevent heart surgery—until the federal government stepped in and stopped this marketing practice.

For now, it's not known whether those increased nitric oxide levels produced by L-arginine translate into reduced risk of heart attack and stroke. I wouldn't take any of these supplements yet—not until we know more about their safety as well as their effectiveness—but stay tuned, because studies are now under way. Until then, you've got another possible reason to take statins or ACE inhibitors if your doctor has prescribed them. Both classes of drugs are known to boost nitric oxide. What else raises nitric oxide? Foods that I've promoted in this chapter: dark chocolate, red wine, oats, and fish oils.

Antioxidant Supplements

One of the key steps in the development of arterial plaque is the oxidation of LDL cholesterol. That's why there's been so much fuss lately over antioxidants, which are food compounds that block oxidation at the cellular levels. Our bodies depend on them to mount a vigorous defense against arteriosclerosis. Now the health stores bristle with antioxidant supplements that claim to offer protection against vascular disease: vitamin C, vitamin E, beta-carotene, lycopene, lutein, selenium, and flavonoids. (I've devoted special consideration elsewhere in this chapter to two other antioxidants: coenzyme Q_{10} and tocotrienols.)

Most of us are accustomed to taking vitamins and minerals. We grew up on chewable multivitamins and were given vitamin C at the first sign of the sniffles. From there, taking vitamin E, the mineral selenium, or any other of these food derivatives may not seem like such a big leap. But don't let your comfort level cloud your judgment. There is no good evidence that any of these supplements reduce your risk of arteriosclerosis. And one of them—beta-carotene—has even been shown to *increase* rates of cancer in people who smoke.

Although antioxidant supplements aren't such a smart idea, you can still put the power of antioxidants to work for you. Decades of scientific research have shown that you can reduce your risk of heart disease and possibly stroke by getting your antioxidants as nature intended: in food. Fruits and vegetables are loaded with them. Look for produce with deeply colored red, yellow, or orange flesh or dark leafy greens. Other fantastic sources of dietary antioxidants are cooked tomatoes, onions, garlic, flaxseeds, red grapes, green tea, nuts, and—my favorite source— dark chocolate.

VITAMIN E PRODUCTS: BEST-SELLERS AREN'T ALWAYS BEST FOR YOU

A few years ago, there were early reports that tocotrienols (antioxidant compounds with vitamin E–like activity) may lower LDL cholesterol. More recent studies are turning up mixed evidence, with some studies showing an LDL reduction of 10 percent or greater—and other studies showing no reduction at all. At the least, tocotrienols are probably fairly harmless, but clinical tests have not provided a dosage for those who want to try them. And if you go shopping for tocotrienols, be aware: their cousin, called gamma-tocopherol and often sold simply as "vitamin E," probably receives more display space in your health store. Don't be fooled into buying it. Gamma tocopherol is known to have absolutely no effect on blood cholesterol!

DHEA (dehydroepiandrosterone)

Your body naturally produces DHEA, a steroid that's used in the production of estrogen and testosterone. Around age 35, levels of DHEA begin to decline. This dropoff has naturally led to speculation that decreased DHEA might be a cause of several age-related problems, including heart disease.

In 1986, a group of California scientists studied a group of 242 retired men and found that those with lower levels of DHEA in their blood were more likely to develop cardiovascular disease. This and other studies sent DHEA supplement sales soaring. Unfortunately, follow-up studies of the retired men did *not* show any continued connection between DHEA and heart problems. Nor were other scientists able to duplicate those early results in subsequent tests.

DHEA *can* help you revisit adolescence, however—by causing acne. Like other steroids, it can also lead to unwanted hair growth. Long-term use can cause breast enlargement in men. And since DHEA is used by the body to manufacture sex hormones, it can raise your risk of breast or prostate cancer. I don't recommend this supplement for heart protection.

Red Yeast Rice Extract (Cholestin)

If you have high cholesterol, it's likely that you take a statin drug such as Pravachol, Zocor, Lipitor, Crestor, or Mevacor. These drugs work, but they are expensive. That's why so many people have turned to red yeast rice extract as a low-cost alternative. One commercial preparation—Cholestin—was particularly popular until the FDA banned its sale in the United Sates.

Cholestin and other red yeast rice products are made by naturally fermenting rice with the *Monascus purpureus* strain of red yeast. Most of us know red yeast rice extract from the red color it lends to many Chinese dishes—including the delicious Peking duck—but it also contains chemicals known as monacolins, which act in a manner similar to pricey statins. In fact, one of the monacolins in Cholestin is identical to lovastatin, which is the active ingredient in the prescription drug Mevacor. Cholestin also contains an artery-friendly trio of sterols (plant fats that absorb cholesterol), isoflavones, and unsaturated fatty acids.

Clinical studies of red yeast rice extract are impressive. Red yeast rice extract has been shown to lower LDL cholesterol anywhere from 13 to 26 percent while raising the HDL cholesterol. It also cuts triglycerides by 13 to 34 percent.

Cholestin found itself at the center of an alt-med storm in 1998. The FDA banned it from health-store shelves on the grounds that one of its ingredients—lovastatin—had already been ruled a prescription drug ingredient for use in Mevacor. The presence of lovastatin made Cholestin an unapproved and illegal drug, not a dietary supplement. Thousands of Americans were outraged, believing that the FDA had acted in the interest of major pharmaceutical companies and yanked an affordable cholesterol treatment out of their hands. Many continue to buy Cholestin in Canada and other countries or to purchase the other red yeast rice extracts available in some health stores. Should you do the same?

Someday that may be the right strategy, but not for now. Here are the top reasons to stick with prescription drugs instead:

1. You can't count on consistent doses of cholesterol-lowering ingredients in red yeast rice extract. Scientists at that other large university in Los Angeles (UCLA) analyzed the monacolin content of nine different red yeast rice preparations. Some products contained up to half of one percent monacolins—and some contained none at all.

2. Only one of the nine products tested at the UCLA lab contained the full range of monacolin compounds that are present in red yeast rice. No one knows yet which monacolins have the best capacity for lowering cholesterol, so by excluding the whole range, these products may be reducing their potency.

3. You could be poisoned. Seven of the nine products tested at UCLA were found to contain citrinin, a by-product that occurs when manufacturers bungle the fermentation process. Citrinin can cause kidney failure.

For now, it's essential that you avoid all red yeast rice extracts. If you absolutely insist on taking them, be aware that they come with some of the same side effects as prescription cholesterol medicines, including muscle pain and impaired liver function. People who take red yeast rice extract must have their liver function monitored by a physician.

Guggulipid

Rolls trippingly off the tongue, doesn't it? Americans are improving their pronunciation of Hindi, thanks to the word-of-mouth reputation of this Ayurvedic supplement. Ayurvedic practitioners and health-store clerks may tell you that guggulipid—an extract of resin from the mukul myrrh tree—binds to the cell receptors involved in cholesterol metabolism. They'll also cite an impressive-sounding fact: in 1987, the Indian government approved guggulipid for lowering blood cholesterol levels.

This is when skepticism really pays off. If you dig around for a little more information, you'll find that many (though not all) studies in India are supported by companies with a financial interest in the outcome. In the first good study of guggulipid conducted *outside* India, 103 participants were given either guggulipid or a placebo for eight weeks. Afterward, the average LDL cholesterol of the placebo group dropped—but the LDL cholesterol of the guggulipid group actually rose slightly. There were also six cases of skin reactions in the guggulipid group.

Sometimes the evidence for alternative medicines is frustratingly difficult to interpret. But on guggulipid, the real science is clear: stay away from this supplement.

Chelation Therapy

Chelation therapy is big business. It's been estimated that half a million people pay for this expensive treatment every year.

The unproven theory behind this practice is that minerals such as calcium, lead, iron, zinc, and magnesium can build up in your body over time and cause all sorts of undesirable medical conditions, including heart disease. For about $4,000 (which is rarely reimbursed by insurance plans), chelation therapy practitioners will infuse a concoction containing an agent called EDTA into your bloodstream. EDTA binds to metals and removes them from your body. Removal of these minerals, goes the argument, can improve heart function and prevent or reverse heart disease.

In a well-designed Canadian study, 84 patients with coronary artery disease received either an infusion of chelation therapy or a placebo twice a week for fifteen weeks and then once every month for three additional months. None of the patients showed any signs of improved heart function.

What's worse is that chelation therapy can actually *cause* heart problems, including arrthymias and cardiac arrest. Other possible side effects include kidney failure, decreased calcium levels, convulsions, prolonged bleeding, and hypotension. This is one therapy you can permanently cross off your list.

The Complete Prescription for Preventing
Heart Attack and Stroke

DAILY STRATEGIES
The Mediterranean and More Diet
Cardiovascular exercise: at least 30 minutes a day, 5 days a week
Fish oils: one serving of fatty fish per week or 1 gram daily of a
     supplement containing both EPA and DHA
Folic acid: 800 micrograms daily from either food or supplements

Mind-body therapies (relaxation, biofeedback, anger management): practice the mind-body therapy of your choice regularly, especially if you have heart disease (though these therapies are good for all of us).

Meditation (only if you enjoy this therapy and feel it has a calming effect): on a daily basis; practice for as long as you need to achieve a peaceful, relaxed state.

Conventional drugs (including enteric-coated baby aspirin): as prescribed

IN SPECIAL CIRCUMSTANCES
(LISTED IN PARENTHESES BELOW)

Gingko biloba (for peripheral artery vascular disease): take 40 to 50 milligrams of a gingko product called EGb 761 (available from German suppliers) or an American gingko extract standardized to 24 percent gingko flavone glycosides and 6 percent terpene lactones.

Hawthorn (as an adjuvant for treating congestive heart failure): HeartCare, to be used only under supervision of a physician. The usual dosage ranges from 80 milligrams twice daily to 160 milligrams three times daily, taken with meals.

Magnesium (only if you live in a soft-water community): 320 milligrams daily

11

Boosting
Brain Function

**WHAT YOUR DOCTOR HASN'T TOLD YOU
AND THE HEALTH-STORE CLERK DOESN'T KNOW
ABOUT ALTERNATIVE MEDICINE FOR BRAIN FUNCTION**

What Your Doctor Hasn't Told You About Alternative Medicine for Brain Function	And What the Health-Store Clerk Doesn't Know
The best way to preserve your mental functioning and prevent Alzheimer's disease can't be ordered at a pharmacy.	This form of brain protection can't be found in a supplement, either.
You may be able to help ward off memory loss and Alzheimer's disease with fish oils.	Which fish oils are best for preserving memory and preventing dementia
Antioxidants may slow the loss of memory.	Why you shouldn't get your antioxidants (especially vitamin E) from pills
As you age, the brain loses its ability to maintain balance.	The cheapest, most pleasurable way to regain lost balancing skills

(continued)

What Your Doctor Hasn't Told You About Alternative Medicine for Brain Function	And What the Health-Store Clerk Doesn't Know
Several studies conclude that gingko biloba leads to sharper memory and concentration.	Several other studies show just the opposite.
Huperzine A may help people with Alzheimer's disease improve their memory.	This supplement is backed by preliminary findings only—and it may interact with conventional treatments for Alzheimer's.
Preliminary studies show that coenzyme Q_{10} may help treat Parkinson's disease.	Why you should take it only under the supervision of a doctor

You'll find much more information about these therapies—as well as many others—in the rest of this chapter.

As the brain ages, several normal changes occur—and not all of them are bad. First and foremost, your short-term memory becomes less reliable. Although long-term memory remains fine, and memories of your first big date or the birth of a child are still fairly fresh, it's not unusual to experience difficulty recalling minor events that have recently taken place. *Where did I put the car keys? What was the chore I was supposed to perform?* I remember how easy it once was for me to remember ten-digit phone numbers I could even carry on a conversation while memorizing a long-distance number. Now, in my sixties, I have to reach for a pad and copy down the number immediately, because my brain just won't store that information the way it used to.

Most people also lose some of their multiprocessor functions as they grow older, which means that it's harder to focus on more than one task at a time. My teenage son, Samuel, can listen to music and e-mail his friends while reading his latest school assignment. By contrast, I can no longer walk down a flight of stairs while letting my brain's attention wander to one of my projects. Instead, I concentrate on the stairs to be sure I don't stumble. Hand-eye coordination and reaction time also slow down. That's why children love to challenge adults to compete with them at video games. The grown-ups usually lose badly.

A lesser-known consequence of brain aging is difficulty with balance. When I was the scientific director of the Buck Institute for Age Research several years ago, we conducted a study of older residents in California's Marin County. We found that the main cause of disability in people age 85 and above (at least in Marin County) was problems with balance. Balance problems can get really serious when they lead to falls and hip fractures, which are a damaging condition for older people. Twenty-five percent of older people who suffer hip fractures do not survive the subsequent twelve months.

But it's important to take a practical view of this situation. First of all, short-term memory, multiprocessing skills, hand-eye coordination, and balance do not instantly vanish when you blow out the candles at your fortieth birthday party. These capabilities diminish gradually, over decades. More important, these changes do not have to alter the quality of your life. Yes, you'll probably notice some age-related brain changes, but the experience that you've acquired over a lifetime more than makes up for any losses. You may not be able to beat your child at a video game, but you know a lot more about how to navigate the challenges that life presents. A few of the skills you enjoy as an adult are those of evaluating conflicting claims and making good decisions based on the information available. You'll need those mental resources if you wander into a health store looking for supplements to boost normal brain function.

In contrast to the normal and gradual losses of mental agility, there are diseases that can deal a serious blow to your brain's function. One of the most common is Alzheimer's disease. The risk of Alzheimer's increases as you get older; by age 85, one out of every three people will develop this devastating disorder. Alzheimer's victims suffer major-league memory gaps and often cannot recall their own addresses, the names of close family members, and other vital pieces of information. Alzheimer's is often preceded by a condition called mild cognitive impairment (MCI), which causes mental impairment that is greater than normal age-related memory lapses but does not seriously hamper daily functioning.

Another brain disorder whose risk grows exponentially with age is Parkinson's disease. In this condition, cells in a region of the brain called the substantia nigra are destroyed. Victims suffer from tremors and uncontrollable movements (usually in their upper extremities), rigidity or stiffness in their limbs, slowness in walking and other tasks, and difficulties with balance. The condition may also involve loss of memory and other brain functions. Although there are medications available to treat Parkinson's, they can be as tough on you as the disease itself.

Both the normal age-related changes in mental function and the higher risk of severe cognitive impairment have led many of us to seek ways to rejuvenate our brains. I recently visited the health store near my office at the university and asked the clerk if anything could reverse memory loss. He handed me a jar and told me that it contained ingredients that would "absolutely" improve my recall. I looked at the label and learned that the product contained gingko biloba along with 45 minerals, nutrients, and vitamins. Gingko, along with several other supplements, has a reputation for sustaining mental agility. Revitalizing brain function is an intriguing prospect, so let's use our experienced adult brains to investigate it further.

Conventional Medications for Brain Function: Little to Offer

Conventional medicine offers no treatment for normal age-related losses in brain functions, and it doesn't have a whole lot more to address the serious cognitive disorders. Currently, the first line of treatment for Alzheimer's disease is made up of two types of drugs. One class of drugs indirectly helps to increase acetylcholine, a brain chemical that appears to affect memory and learning, and the other group decreases the influence of another brain chemical, glutamate. These drugs include donepezil (Aricept), galantamine (Reminyl), rivastigmine (Exelon), and memantine (Namenda). None of these drugs is a cure. They appear to work best for people in the early or middle stages of Alzheimer's. At best, these drugs can only slow the progression of Alzheimer's, and some of them can cause a host of problems, including nausea, vomiting, and liver failure.

There is mounting evidence that inflammation may also play a role in brain aging and possibly increase the risk of Alzheimer's disease. Preliminary studies indicate that statins—the same drugs that lower cholesterol—may have anti-inflammatory effects that could prevent Alzheimer's. Until statins have more conclusive evidence under their belt, no one should take statins for the sole reason of warding off brain disease. But if you're already taking statins to prevent heart problems, consider these medications as possible bonus protection against Alzheimer's.

Several years ago, hormone replacement therapy was promoted to prevent Alzheimer's disease (along with just about every other problem associated with aging) in menopausal women. However, the most recent findings of the Women's Health Initiative indicate that estrogen replacement therapy—either alone or with progestin—does not reduce the risk of dementia.

The current drugs for Parkinson's disease are aimed at reducing symptoms such as tremor and rigidity. Unfortunately, they also have serious side effects and do little to slow the progression of the underlying disease.

To Slow Aging, Stay Active

I spent ten years working with some of the world's greatest scientists on the MacArthur Foundation Study of Successful Aging. We selected a group of 70-year-olds who appeared to be in good physical and mental health and then followed them for the next ten years to document how well they maintained their health status. We were particularly interested in the subjects who maintained their cognitive vigor—and were surprised to find that the folks who stayed the sharpest were the ones who remained the most physically active.

It's not yet clear just how exercise might maintain good brain health. But there is evidence that physical activity stimulates the brain chemicals necessary for effective functioning. Animal studies also back up the effectiveness of exercise for preserving brain function. Cardiovascular activity and weight training boast another benefit: they help you maintain your balance and reduce your risk of falls. (For maximum effectiveness, weight training for balance should focus on strengthening your hips and legs, though you shouldn't neglect your other muscle groups.)

So protect your aging brain (even if you're still fairly young) and find ways to stay active for life. If arthritis or back problems are preventing you from working out, don't assume that you just have to live with the pain. Good treatments for these conditions are available—and important, because you'll need to get physically active to stay mentally sharp. Check out my suggestions elsewhere in this book for easing the pain of joint and back problems.

Many people, including several eminent scientists, believe that to prevent brain decline, it's not just physical activity that counts—it's important to keep up mental activity as well. While I have not found a convincing body of scientific research to support this claim, my clinical experience with older people is that those who feed their brains are the most likely to retain their mental functions. So include some challenging intellectual activities in your daily schedule. Solve crossword puzzles, volunteer to teach a skill to others, or play strategy games like bridge or chess.

You can also counter the decline in short-term memory that occurs with aging by learning a few new tricks. There are courses in tuning up your memory, and there are a number of books that can help you. I recommend a book called *The Memory Prescription,* by Gary Small, who is the director of UCLA's Center on Aging.

The Discriminating Consumer's Guide to Alternative Medicine for Healthy Brain Function

As you may have suspected, there are no magic bullets to reverse memory loss or other cognitive problems. Not in the pharmacy—and not in the aisles of the health stores. Does that mean you have to sit at home with your hands folded neatly in your lap and accept the inevitable decline? No. A few forms of alternative medicine offer real protection against memory and balance loss; there is also hope for victims of serious cognitive impairment.

HIGHLY RECOMMENDED ALTERNATIVE THERAPIES FOR BOOSTING BRAIN FUNCTION

Fish oils (omega-3 fatty acids)
If you're not yet eating fish (or taking a fish-oil supplement) to reduce your risk of heart disease, depression, and possibly cancer, perhaps this will persuade you: fish oils appear to have a protective effect against Alzheimer's disease and memory loss. In a Dutch study of 815 healthy

older people, those who consumed fish at least once a week were 60 percent less likely to develop Alzheimer's than people who ate fish less frequently. These results held true even when other risk factors were ruled out. And we know that Dutch senior citizens who eat plenty of fish show less cognitive impairment than their counterparts.

Another study tracked 3,718 Chicago residents age 65 and older. The researchers found that those who ate fish two times a week slowed their mental decline by 13 percent per year.

DOSAGE: Eat one or two servings of fatty fish weekly, or buy a fish-oil supplement and take 1 gram per day. When taking fish oils specifically for brain health, I recommend finding a supplement that contains at least 50 percent DHA (docosahexaenoic acid), as there is a strong link between DHA and brain function. Side effects of fish-oil supplements include gastrointestinal complaints, increased bleeding, and unpleasant breath. For more information about fish and fish oils, see chapter 10, "Preventing Heart Disease and Stroke."

Tai Chi

In the 1990s, the National Institute on Aging solicited scientists to find new ways to help people keep their balance as long as possible. In an acclaimed study by scientists at Emory University in Atlanta, 200 older men and women with an average age of 76 were randomly assigned to one of three groups. The first group spent fifteen weeks undergoing daily tai chi sessions. The second group received balance training, using computerized balance equipment, and the third set was educated in balance and fall prevention. In the four-month period after training, the subjects were monitored for their number of falls. The folks who received balance training and fall-prevention education fell down about as often as they had before the study—but the people who took tai chi cut their number of falls in half.

Tai chi was first developed in China as a martial art. Most practitioners today employ tai chi simply as a series of slow, gentle movements. If you've seen people doing tai chi in a local park or gym, you might have wondered how something that looks so easy can qualify as exercise. Although it's not a cardiovascular workout, tai chi requires a high level of concentration and involves coordination of most of the body's muscles, including those you might not ordinarily use when exercising. I became a fan of tai chi when the board of counselors at my school invited Scott Cole, a well-known tai chi instructor, to our annual retreat. Standing on the front lawn of a resort hotel, we took off our shoes and followed Scott through tai chi's graceful motions. One of these moves was a gradual transfer of weight from one leg to the other, until the entire body weight was supported on one leg. Again, this activity may sound like a piece of cake, but it was both mentally and physically challenging. And by the end of the hour, I could sense an improvement in my balance and a new lightness to my step. Tai chi can confer its benefits on anyone—even younger people will appreciate its meditative, relaxing quality—but it's especially useful for those folks whose painful joints or limited mobility keeps them from participating in other more strenuous activities.

Antioxidants (Dietary)

Here's yet another reason to eat well: studies indicate that dietary consumption of certain antioxidants can protect your memory. In one study of 422 Swiss residents age 65 to 94, high blood levels of vitamin C and beta-carotene (both are antioxidants) were linked to good performance on tests of free recall, recognition, and vocabulary. Does this mean that you can sharpen your brain by taking supplements of vitamin C and beta-carotene? Apparently not. The subjects in this study received their daily dose of these antioxidants mainly from the fruits and vegetables in their diets, not from pills.

Although the Swiss study showed no relation between vitamin E (another antioxidant) and retention of memory, other evidence suggests that it's a good idea to include vitamin E in your diet. When researchers at the Rush Institute for Healthy Aging and the Rush Alzheimer's Disease

Center followed 800 older Chicagoans for four years, dietary vitamin E was associated with a reduced risk of Alzheimer's disease—although this occurred only in people who were genetically predisposed to the disease in the first place. This finding is bolstered by the National Health and Nutrition Examination Survey, which discovered that people whose blood levels of vitamin E decreased over a period of six years were more likely to suffer from poor memory.

DOSAGE: To boost the odds of retaining your memory, make sure to increase your antioxidant load by eating plenty of fruits and vegetables, as well as nuts and seeds for vitamin E. Don't take a vitamin E supplement, as the data do not support its use.

VITAMIN E, WHERE ARE YOU?

According to the Centers for Disease Control and Prevention, nearly 30 percent of adult Americans have low blood levels of vitamin E. This group may be at increased risk for Alzheimer's disease as well as heart disease and some cancers. Vitamin E supplements have performed poorly in clinical trials, suggesting that it's far better to get your daily dose of E through your diet. That's not easy to do, as there are only a few foods—mainly nuts and seeds—that are high in vitamin E. Fortunately, nuts and seeds are incredibly tasty. Toast them lightly and toss them in salads or cereals, or enjoy them straight out of the bag for a filling snack.

RECOMMENDED ALTERNATIVE TREATMENTS FOR BOOSTING BRAIN FUNCTION

Coenzyme Q_{10} (Ubiquinone) (for Parkinson's disease only)
It is hypothesized that in Parkinson's disease, part of the brain is attacked by free radicals. This has led to speculation that coenzyme Q_{10}, a

natural substance that protects the cells against oxidative damage, might help slow or halt the progress of Parkinson's disease. In 2002, the National Institutes of Health funded a trial of coenzyme Q_{10} on people in the early stages of Parkinson's. After sixteen months of treatment, patients who'd received the highest doses (1200 milligrams daily) of coenzyme Q_{10} saw a significant decrease in disability when compared with patients who took a placebo. A German study of 28 patients found a similar reduction in early Parkinson's symptoms with coenzyme Q_{10}. These results provide some hope that coenzyme Q_{10} may play a role in symptom relief for Parkinson's patients, but larger studies need to be conducted before we know for sure.

Given the serious nature of Parkinson's disease and the relative lack of serious side effects for coenzyme Q_{10}, you might consider a trial of this compound. Use it as an adjunct to conventional treatment and only with your physician's knowledge and guidance.

DOSAGE: 1200 milligrams of coenzyme Q_{10} daily. Side effects of short-term use are rare and include diarrhea, rash, and photophobia (extreme sensitivity to light). This supplement has never been tested for use over long durations, but some of you may decide to accept this risk of the unknown when weighed against the well-documented effects of Parkinson's and the side effects of current medications. Remember to consult with your doctor before using Q_{10} for Parkinson's disease.

Huperzine A (Huperzia serrata)
(for Alzheimer's disease and MCI only)

Thirty million years ago, club mosses were the major component of forests worldwide. Today their existence is limited mostly to tropical and subtropical rain forests, but that hasn't kept one variety of club moss, *Huperzia serrata,* from becoming a popular herbal medicine. It's sold both in China (where it is a component of the Chinese herbal mixture qian ceng ta) and in the West. In the United States, club moss extract is sold under the name huperzine A and is marketed to improve memory loss. There's logic behind this use of club moss, as I'll explain below.

Like the first-line conventional drugs for Alzheimer's disease, huperzine A is known to inhibit the enzyme acetylcholinesterase. The suppression of this enzyme leads to an increase in the brain chemical acetylcholine. And laboratory tests have shown that huperzine A, an antioxidant, protects the brain from damage. Now for the big question: Does huperzine A slow down the progression of Alzheimer's disease?

Soon we'll have an answer. Chinese studies have concluded that huperzine A improves memory—but as you know, I prefer to base my recommendations on studies performed in Western countries, where the scientific review process is usually more rigorous. Luckily, the results of the Chinese studies have ignited the curiosity of American researchers, and now several medical centers in the United States, with a grant from the National Institute on Aging, are testing the effects of huperzine A on Alzheimer's disease as part of a federally funded study.

DOSAGE AND SIDE EFFECTS: Although studies on huperzine A are still in their infancy, Alzheimer's disease is such a serious illness that people with this disorder or its precursor, mild cognitive impairment, might wish to consider using this supplement—but only as an adjunct to conventional treatment and only under the advice of a physician. Because huperzine A appears to act on some of the same neural pathways as prescription cholinesterase inhibitors, your doctor or pharmacist may need to adjust your doses of the conventional drugs. Optimal doses of huperzine A remain unknown, although the current federal study is reviewing twice-daily doses of 200 micrograms and 400 micrograms. The known side effects of huperzine A include nausea and dizziness. Long-term studies of this supplement may uncover other problems—though you may be willing to tolerate this uncertainty when it is weighed against the frightening effects of Alzheimer's.

ACCEPTABLE ALTERNATIVE TREATMENTS FOR
BOOSTING BRAIN FUCTION

Gingko biloba

It's estimated that 4.6 million Americans take gingko biloba, making it comparable in usage to the twentieth-most-popular prescription drug sold in the United States.

No wonder. The gingko biloba tree is one of the world's oldest, and its extract has been used in Chinese herbal remedies for at least four millennia. It's often used as an all-purpose tonic, which explains why people take it for everything from heart problems to fatigue. But its most popular application is for improved mental function—hence its inclusion in the "brain health" supplement I found in the health store.

There's no shortage of studies on the effect of gingko on normal individuals, although these studies have produced contrasting results. Some have showed significant improvement in memory, while others have shown no benefit over a placebo. In one of the best of these trials (published in the *Journal of the American Medical Association*), 230 healthy volunteers took either gingko or a placebo for six weeks. At the end of the test period, researchers found no difference between the two groups on tests of memory, learning, attention, and concentration.

Gingko has also been tested as a remedy for Alzheimer's disease. In 1997, scientists from the New York Institute for Medical Research published a study (also in the *Journal of the American Medical Association*) showing that Alzheimer's disease progressed less rapidly in patients who took gingko than those receiving a placebo. Unfortunately, no one else has been able to duplicate these results. A more recent trial in the Netherlands of 214 people with dementia (most dementia is caused by Alzheimer's disease) or impaired memory did not find any significant difference between gingko and a placebo.

DOSAGE: Gingko's effects remain unclear, but the leaf extract is fairly safe. (Avoid gingko fruit, which can produce serious allergic reactions. Also, anyone with a history of seizures should not take gingko.) The usual dosage of gingko biloba extract is 120 to 160 milligrams daily, divided into two or three doses. Note that this dosage refers specifically to a concentrated gingko extract known as EGb 761. This extract is manufactured by the German company Schwabe and contains 24 percent glycosides and 6 percent terpenes. This gingko product—and only this gingko product—is approved by Germany's Kommission E and is the extract used in most clinical and laboratory studies of gingko. However, it can be difficult to find EGb 761 in the United States. Although there are many American companies that sell gingko biloba extracts that are standardized to the same amounts of glycosides and terpenes, it is not clear whether these ingredients are the same as those used in the German product. Once again, the federal government's hands are tied when it comes to regulation of herbal products—but it's consumers who feel the pain.

Phosphatidylserine (PS)

Phosphatidylserine (also called PS) is promoted as a cure for age-related memory impairment. Why are health-store clerks so excited about this supplement? For one, phosphatidylserine is a phospholipid that your brain needs to maintain its smooth functioning. (Abnormal phospholipids, caused by genetic disorders, usually cause brain damage.) PS also activates an enzyme called protein kinase C, which plays a key role in memory.

But for all its importance in the brain, PS does not appear to have much effect on memory when taken as a supplement. Many clinical trials have been performed on patients with age-related memory impairment and Alzheimer's disease, with some results showing a slight improvement in word recall and others showing hardly any benefit at all. The only upside? PS has few side effects.

DOSAGE: 100 milligrams, taken twice daily.

DO NOT USE THESE ALTERNATIVE TREATMENTS FOR BOOSTING BRAIN FUNCTION

Vinpocetine

Vinpocetine is an herbal remedy derived from the periwinkle plant. This product was developed in Hungary and is promoted in the United States to increase brain function. I'm intrigued by preliminary studies of vinpocetine, which show some improvement in memory, attention, and concentration, but high doses can cause a drop in blood pressure. Further studies are needed to confirm that vinpocetine's benefits outweigh its risks.

Acetyl-N-carnitine

Often packaged inside so-called brain-power supplements, the amino acid acetyl-N-carnitine has shown some beneficial effects on thyroid disease, Peyronie's disease, and patients on dialysis. But there is insufficient evidence to recommend it now for improving memory or brain function.

CDP-Choline (Citicholine)

For more than twenty-five years, doctors have tried using CDP-choline—a substance thought to have a protective effect on cell membranes—to improve memory in disorders affecting brain function, including Alzheimer's disease. Indeed, an assessment of thirteen well-controlled trials published in *The Cochrane Database of Systematic Reviews* showed that choline has a modest but positive effect on memory and behavior.

There's a hitch. In most of these studies, choline was given by injection into the veins or muscles. This delivery method is both difficult and costly. And the longest study lasted for only three months, which isn't enough time to establish the potential side effects. Given that choline has yielded only small results (it certainly didn't cure anyone), I do not recommend it at this time.

The Complete Prescription for Boosting Brain Function

Tai chi: 30 minutes daily

Fish-oil supplements containing EPA and DHA: 1 gram daily

Cardiovascular exercise: 30 minutes daily, at least five days a week

Weight training (to compensate for balance problems): two to three
times weekly

Fruits and vegetables: five to nine servings daily

Nuts and seeds: at least one portion a day

Challenging intellectual activity: daily

Coenzyme Q_{10} (for Parkinson's disease only): as prescribed by a
physician and only as an adjunct to conventional treatment

Huperzine A (for Alzheimer's disease and MCI only): as prescribed
by a physician and only as an adjunct to conventional treatment;
your doctor may need to adjust the doses of prescription
cholinesterase inhibitors.

12

Cancer Prevention
and Treatment

WHAT YOUR DOCTOR HASN'T TOLD YOU
AND THE HEALTH-STORE CLERK DOESN'T KNOW
ABOUT ALTERNATIVE MEDICINE FOR CANCER

What Your Doctor Hasn't Told You About Alternative Medicine for Cancer	And What the Health-Store Clerk Doesn't Know
Antioxidants may cut your risk of cancer.	The best way to reap the benefits of antioxidants
In test tubes, shark cartilage slows the cancer-related growth of blood vessels.	Whether shark cartilage has any effects in real life
According to laboratory analyses, mistletoe contains proteins that appear to slow cancer.	Whether mistletoe has the same effect outside of the petri dish
Several herbs can slow the growth of prostate cancer cells . . . in the laboratory.	Whether these herbs are safe and effective for male cancer patients
	(continued)

What Your Doctor Hasn't Told You About Alternative Medicine for Cancer	And What the Health-Store Clerk Doesn't Know
Acupuncture relieves nausea and vomiting caused by chemotherapy.	Which form of acupuncture is most effective and how long its effects last
You'll find much more information about these therapies—as well as many others—in the rest of this chapter.	

When I was an administrator at the National Institutes of Health, a controversy erupted over Laetrile, a compound derived from apricot pits. The physician who first produced Laetrile claimed that it was a newly discovered vitamin—he called it "B_{17},"—and blamed most cancers on a deficiency of this very substance. By taking Laetrile, he argued, people could cure their cancer. The federal government disagreed on all counts and blocked its sale.

For decades, the battle raged. Even as people offered passionate testimony that Laetrile had cured or slowed their cancer, federal agents arrested anyone who tried to sell Laetrile in the United States. Many cancer patients were confused: why, they wondered, would their government ignore a potential treatment for their disease? Some desperate folks—including the actor Steve McQueen—went all the way to Tijuana to buy the stuff.

As I watched the debate escalate, I wondered why the government didn't take the obvious step of performing a good clinical trial of Laetrile. Finally, in 1980, they did exactly this. The study concluded that Laetrile had absolutely no effect on tumor growth and that one of its metabolic by-products is the deadly poison cyanide. Almost overnight, public interest in the supplement dried up, with a few exceptions. Twenty-five years later, Laetrile is still advertised on the Web for sale in other countries, proving that shady cancer treatments never die—they just move offshore. Perhaps the only good to come out of the Laetrile disaster is that the NIH learned their lesson, and now popular "cures" for cancer no longer go ignored; instead, they are tested quickly.

I don't blame the cancer patients who tried Laetrile, although they put their lives in further jeopardy by doing so. When cancer is diagnosed, fear and confusion make it difficult to come to good conclusions about alternative medicine. Well-meaning family members and friends who urge their favored therapies on the cancer patient unwittingly add to the problem.

This chapter is here to dispel this confusion and make some of your tough decisions a little easier. Although there aren't any alternative therapies that appear to reverse or slow cancer's progress, there are several that can reduce your suffering and return a welcome measure of control to your life.

For those of you who are hoping to prevent cancer, the news brightens. By strengthening your daily commitment to good health habits, you can mount your best defense against this killer. This chapter gives you the details you need about how much exercise is necessary, which foods prevent certain cancers, and which popular cancer-prevention supplements aren't worth the time it takes to pop them.

Conventional Medicine: Know Your Odds

Cancer is the term for a group of diseases characterized by abnormal cell growth. Conventional therapies include surgery to remove the cancer (when possible) and chemicals, radiation, or hormones to slow or kill the growth of cancer when surgery is not a good option. Each of these treatments is intended to remove the existing cancer and to prevent a dangerous stage of cancer known as metastasis, in which cancerous cells travel to other parts of the body and destroy vital organs and tissues.

The success rate of conventional treatments varies widely. Some cancers have a nearly 100 percent cure rate; others are almost always terminal. Unfortunately, chemotherapy and radiation kill normal cells as well as tumor cells, and they can have severe side effects that include fatigue, nausea, loss of appetite, and hair loss. That's why so many of us are excited about new cancer treatments on the horizon. These innovative treatments involve biologic agents that are specific to the type of cancer being treated, and they hold great promise for better results and fewer side effects. How far you carry current conventional treatment for cancer is a decision best made with your doctor. This decision should factor in the likelihood of success and the severity of side effects.

Cancer Prevention: The Power Is in Your Hands

Sometimes we fall into the trap of believing that cancer is a kind of grim lottery and that there's nothing you can do to determine whether your number will be called. Sadly enough, sometimes that's true. But in fact, 60 percent of all cancers are preventable. By making wise lifestyle choices, you can stop cancer before it starts.

First of all, if you smoke . . . quit. Now. Smoking is the primary cause of lung cancer, one of the deadliest of diseases, and can also lead to cancers of the mouth, tongue, throat, and bladder. Safe sex, in addition to being a safeguard against HIV contamination, can also help protect you against cervical cancer.

Beyond these basics, regular exercise is one of your best tools for cancer prevention. Large-scale studies have shown that even moderate exercise slashes your risk of breast and colon cancers. By walking, hiking, cycling, swimming, or engaging in other activities, you're engaging in a protective strategy more potent than any of the so-called cancer-prevention supplements on the market. Exercise also helps you maintain a healthy weight, which reduces the risk of postmenopausal breast cancer, as well as cancers of the colon, uterus, esophagus, gallbladder, pancreas, and kidney.

Many scientists believe that the first step toward cancer development is the oxidation process caused by free radicals, destructive molecules that wreak havoc throughout your body. Luckily, a defense against free radicals can be found in your backyard garden: many fruits and vegetables contain antioxidants, which are food compounds that stop free radicals in their tracks. By following a diet packed with produce, you may dramatically improve your odds against cancer.

PROSTATE CANCER PREVENTION

In the Nutritional Prevention of Cancer Study, investigators set out to learn the effect of the antioxidant selenium on the recurrence of melanoma. The study's authors found little effect on skin cancer, but they did notice a whopping 65 percent decline in the incidence of prostate cancer in men who took selenium supplements. Other studies have also shown an inverse relationship between the amount of selenium in a man's body and his risk of prostate cancer. Selenium supplements appear to reduce cancer risk only when taken by men whose selenium levels were low to begin with, however. Thanks to food-distribution patterns, selenium deficiency is rarely a problem in the United States, especially among people who are adequately nourished.

DOSAGE: High doses of selenium can be toxic and produce gastrointestinal problems, nail-bed changes, hair loss, fatigue, and neurological problems, so I don't recommend taking selenium in supplement form. If you want to get more selenium in your diet—which is almost always a safer proposition than taking a pill—try eating Brazil nuts. They contain a whopping 544 micrograms of selenium per ounce, which is almost ten times the recommended daily allowance. (No need to worry about overdosing on Brazil nuts. People rarely get into trouble by consuming high levels of vitamins and minerals in foods.)

More on the importance of vegetables: we know that people who eat very few vegetables have double the risk of colon cancer. It's also clear that a diet high in lycopene, an antioxidant found in cooked tomatoes, is associated with a lower risk of prostate cancer. There's yet another benefit to raising your veggie quotient: you'll automatically increase your intake of fiber. Although there are no crystal-clear links between fiber consumption and colon cancer, societies that consume the most fiber also boast the lowest rates of colon cancer. To lower my own risk of all cancers, I make sure my dinner plate is piled high with vegetables from the carotenoid family (these are the vegetables that are colored yellow, orange, red, or dark green on the inside) and tomato products such as tomato paste and red sauces. I also enjoy green tea, soybeans, garlic, and cruciferous vegetables like cauliflower. The antioxidant levels of these foods make them a smart bet for the educated diner.

POPULAR . . . BUT UNPROVEN

According to a survey by UCLA's Center for Human Nutrition and School of Medicine, here are the herbal supplements cancer patients turn to most often:

- astragalus (huang qi)
- cat's claw
- mistletoe
- saw palmetto
- milk thistle
- shiitake mushrooms

Despite what you may hear, none of these supplements has been proven to successfully fight cancer.

With the exception of selenium discussed in the box on page 219, note that studies have failed to show any cancer-preventing benefit for antioxidants when they are taken as supplements. (For more information about antioxidant supplements, see page 229, later in this chapter.) You'd also do well to cut back on red meat. A number of epidemiological studies have linked the consumption of red meat to an increased risk of cancer. For example, one study showed that people who ate beef four or more times a week were more than twice as likely to develop stomach cancer than those who ate less beef. In the same study, people who preferred their meat barbecued, well done, or fried were at a higher risk for cancers of the pancreas, colon, and breast. One theory behind this meat-and-cancer association is that cooked meats produce heterocyclic amines, which are cancer-causing agents.

The Discriminating Consumer's Guide to Cancer Alternatives

If you have cancer, your first-line therapy should be conventional medicine. Delaying proper therapy could have deadly results. Once you and your doctor have agreed on a course of treatment, you can turn to alternatives as an adjunct source of help. Alternative medicine can fill a long-empty niche in cancer therapy, as a reliever of discomfort caused by both the illness and the treatment.

HIGHLY RECOMMENDED ALTERNATIVE TREATMENTS FOR CANCER

Exercise
Although exercise is not a cancer cure, scientists have known for decades that it can lift the fatigue associated with chemotherapy and ra-

diation therapy. In one particularly promising study in the journal *Cancer,* patients who had undergone high-dose chemotherapy and stem-cell transplantation were put through a six-week physical training program. At the end of the program, they demonstrated more energy and higher scores on tests of physical performance. This was good news for the patients, but not really surprising. The best news was this: After completing the exercise program, the patients had higher blood counts, suggesting that exercise may help battle the cancer as well.

Of course, it can be difficult to exercise when you're tired in the first place. Try for 30 minutes of activity, 5 days a week—but don't let this recommendation become an additional source of stress if you find it impossible to follow. Just do as much as you reasonably can. Even a few minutes a day may help.

Folic Acid and Calcium

Epidemiological studies link high consumption of calcium and folic acid to lower rates of colon cancer. Just how calcium and folic acid might ward off colon cancer is unknown, but since both supplements also offer well-documented protection from other chronic conditions such as osteoporosis and heart disease, it's certainly smart for everyone to take them.

DOSAGE: Get 1000 to 1500 milligrams of calcium daily from diet and supplements, and make sure to get 800 micrograms of folic acid a day from diet and supplements. For proper calcium absorption, you'll also need vitamin D. You can obtain this vitamin by getting a few minutes of sun on your unprotected arms and face a couple of times each week. You can also take 1000 IU daily of vitamin D if sun exposure isn't possible; take supplements of D in the winter if you get sun exposure but live in a climate where the sun's rays are weak.

Massage

Massage won't cure cancer, but there are several good reasons to use it anyway: massage relieves anxiety, promotes relaxation, and may assist in pain management. If your illness or treatment has left you feeling divorced from your body, massage can you help you regain a sense of wholeness.

One form of massage, called manual lymph drainage, has a more direct therapeutic use for some cancer patients. This massage treatment relieves swelling in the arms, a common side effect of mastectomy surgery. Major surgery for pelvic cancer can bring on leg swelling; massage may be helpful in this circumstance as well.

You may have heard that massage can spread cancer throughout your body. There's no evidence to prove that massage has such an effect, but stay on the safe side and hire an experienced therapist who will avoid the site of the tumor. Take special care if you have bony metastasis (cancer that's spread to the bones)—because fractures might occur—or if either the cancer or the therapy causes you to bleed easily. All cancer patients should avoid deep abdominal massage, which might lead to internal bleeding.

Group Therapy and Emotional Support

In 1989, headlines delivered the astonishing news: breast-cancer patients who regularly attended group therapy experienced longer survival rates than those who didn't. What you may not have heard is that later investigators were unable to replicate these good results. Perhaps that's because more traditional breast-cancer treatments have improved in the last quarter-century (some have incorporated group therapy) and extended survival rates on their own.

There remain excellent reasons to join a support group designed especially for cancer patients, no matter what kind of cancer you're facing. Group therapy contributes to healing—in the sense that healing involves the mind and spirit as well as the body—by decreasing stress, anxiety, pain, and depression. If you dislike the idea of joining a group, that's fine, but know this: people who feel pessimistic or resigned to their fate upon receiving a cancer diagnosis can learn via support and therapy to develop a more positive fighting spirit.

Acupuncture

If you suffer from nausea and vomiting as a result of cancer treatment, you might want to try acupuncture. A well-designed study published in the *Journal of the American Medical Association* (*JAMA*) found that acupuncture offers excellent relief from these symptoms. It may also help control pain associated with cancer and chemotherapy, although the evidence for this use isn't as strong.

Of the various forms of acupuncture available, electroacupuncture (also known as Western acupuncture, in which mild electrical stimulation is applied to the needles) appears to be the most powerful against nausea and vomiting.

In the *JAMA* study, cancer patients received electroacupuncture treatment once daily for five days as they were undergoing chemotherapy. You may or may not need such intensive treatment. Bear in mind that the nausea relief is only temporary—after nine days, all good effects appear to fade—so you'll need to time your visits to the acupuncturist accordingly.

Hypnosis

In a review of six clinical trials, hypnosis was more effective against cancer pain than conventional treatments. This is good news for people who dislike the strong side effects of pain medications or who find them of limited use.

RECOMMENDED ALTERNATIVE TREATMENTS FOR CANCER

Mind-Body Therapies

I once gave a talk at a meeting where Bernie Siegel, M.D., was also on the bill. Dr. Siegel gave a wonderfully uplifting talk about his Exceptional Cancer Patient program, which sends its participants through group and individual therapies designed to use the mind as a healing tool. He left me—and the rest of his audience—more convinced than ever of the mind's ability to perform impressive feats. Unfortunately, when a study looked at survival rates for people enrolled in the Exceptional Cancer Patient program and then compared them with matched control groups, it found no difference between the two. This doesn't reduce my enthusiasm for Dr. Siegel's compassionate healing abilities. But not everyone with cancer can enlist the aid of a Dr. Siegel.

Other mind-body therapies—such as relaxation, hypnosis (whose pain-relieving powers are discussed separately in this chapter), yoga, and meditation—also do not appear to have clear-cut curative powers, yet the evidence we do have is tantalizing. In a 2002 review of mind-body therapies, about half of the good clinical trials showed an increased survival rate. The other 50 percent showed little or no change. From a dispassionately scientific standpoint, those results are inconclusive. But mind-body treatments are so safe that most of us would be willing to take our chances on them.

Even if mind-body therapies never prove themselves as true cancer fighters, they are a smart supplement to conventional treatment. In a 2004 study published in the journal *Psychoneuroendocrinology,* patients with cancer of the breast and prostate participated in an eight-week program of relaxation, meditation, and yoga. At the end of the study, the patients reported better sleep, less stress, and improved overall quality of life.

This study had some drawbacks. There was no placebo and no control group. But its results suggest that by learning a few easy and inexpensive techniques, you can reduce the stress and suffering associated with cancer diagnosis and treatment. Other studies of relaxation, meditation, and hypnosis have further shown that mind-body therapies can reduce cancer-related pain.

At a time when you may feel helpless—and therefore more vulnerable to the immune-suppressing effects of depression—mind-body therapies also increase positive feelings of working against the cancer. So practice yoga, relax, meditate, or engage in whatever mind-body therapy you most enjoy. Consider it a prescription for well-being in a time of crisis. (Other methods of healing, such as therapeutic touch, Reiki, faith healing, and prayer have less evidence behind them, even as adjuncts to conventional medicine.)

You can find instructions for the relaxation response, a popular relaxation and meditation technique, on pages 19–20. Many hospitals offer yoga classes designed especially for people with cancer and other chronic illnesses.

Fish Oils (omega-3 fatty acids)

By eating a serving of fatty fish once or twice a week, you can protect your heart and help ward off stroke. Now there is preliminary evidence that the omega-3 fatty acids found in cold-water fish may also be a useful adjunct to cancer treatment. Researchers at Louisiana State University found that fish oils slowed tumor growth in laboratory mice and rats. It's too early to assume that humans will have the same positive response, but I'm heartened by a study showing that breast-cancer patients who consumed higher levels of omega-3s had an improved response to chemotherapy. Still, there's no definitive proof that fish oils can fight cancer in humans. You've got plenty of other reasons to enjoy salmon or tuna, however, so why not put these fish on your weekly menu? You can also choose to take a fish-oil supplement instead, especially if your appetite is weak or if you're concerned about mercury contamination.

DOSAGE: One or two servings of fatty fish per week or 1 gram daily of a fish-oil supplement containing both EPA (eicosapentaenoic acid) and DHA (docosahexanoic acid).

Aromatherapy

Inhaling the essential oils of flowers or herbs can promote comfort and ease. Cancer therapists and hospice workers appreciate scents such as lavender, sandalwood, and bergamot because they are inexpensive and easy to administer, and have few side effects other than allergic responses.

Aromatherapy oils can be purchased at specialty stores and usually cost less than $10 a vial. You can simply open the top and inhale the scent of fresh herbs or flowers, or you can try my favorite application: add a few drops to massage oil and have your massage therapist apply it directly to your skin as you get a relaxing rubdown. One analysis of several clinical studies showed that massage combined with aromatherapy is more effective than either alone at reducing anxiety and increasing a sense of well-being.

You also have every right to reject aromatherapy if it doesn't suit you. It doesn't matter whether your spouse or friend is comforted by scent; what matters is whether this treatment carries a little stress out of your life.

ACCEPTABLE ALTERNATIVE TREATMENTS FOR CANCER

Guided Imagery

Guided imagery incorporates a wide range of techniques from simple visualization to complex storytelling. Once believed to fight off cancer by stimulating the body's immune response, guided imagery is now usually employed for "softer" purposes, such as relaxation, symptom relief, and coping with the stress of cancer treatment.

No well-conducted studies have proven guided imagery to work against cancer and its symptoms. Nevertheless, guided imagery remains a safe way to relax and perhaps feel more in control of treatment. If you wish to try guided imagery, you can buy one of the many recordings that will walk you through the process (or check one out from the library). You can also hire a professional to help you use guided imagery for the most relaxing effects. Beware, however, of anyone who advertises that he or she can cure cancer with this treatment.

Homeopathy

The most commonly used homeopathic remedy for treatment of cancer is *Arnica montana*. This plant-derived remedy supposedly reduces muscle and tissue trauma.

There is simply no evidence available for *Arnica montana* or other homeopathic treatments for cancer, though homeopathic remedies are very safe if you wish to try them. You are most likely to harness a soothing placebo effect if you're willing to spend the money for an individual consultation with a skilled, compassionate homeopath. Just be sure that you don't let any good feelings from a one-on-one homeopathic session deter you from conventional treatment.

Macrobiotic Diets

Macrobiotic diets are a popular alternative treatment for cancer, perhaps because their highly restrictive nature helps patients feel they are taking appropriately drastic measures in a time of crisis. Although there is no single macrobiotic diet, most versions are vegetarian and very low in fat, with an emphasis on consuming whole grains and soy. You may hear plenty of moving testimonies from people who claim that macrobiotics cured their cancer, but there is little hard evidence. Only two studies of macrobiotic diets for cancer have been conducted, and both of these were seriously flawed. There have been no rigorously controlled studies of macrobiotic diets.

Many people assume that macrobiotic diets, even if not proven, are at least safe. After all, doctors have been begging us to eat low-fat meals for years. They are probably not very dangerous at all—but do inform your physician about your new diet, just to make sure that its radical restrictions won't interfere with your therapy.

Shiitake Mushrooms

Shiitakes supposedly stimulate the function of killer T cells and thus fight cancer. Although there is no good evidence to support this claim, it certainly can't hurt you to enjoy shiitake mushrooms in soups, salads, and other dishes—as long as you don't bust your budget on these expensive treats.

DO NOT USE THESE ALTERNATIVE TREATMENTS FOR CANCER

Antioxidant Supplements

It's been theorized that cancer development begins with the generation of free radicals, highly reactive molecules that can initiate destruction at the cellular level. Antioxidants are food-based chemicals that neutralize free radicals, so it's understandable that many people turn to antioxidant supplements for cancer prevention and treatment. Antioxidant supplements include vitamins A, C, and E, as well as lycopene, beta-carotene, coenzyme Q_{10}, and selenium.

Before you pop an antioxidant pill, be aware that there is considerable debate over the role of antioxidants in cancer prevention and therapy. Proponents have included the venerable two-time Nobel laureate Linus Pauling, who promoted vitamin C to improve immune function and fight cancer. We're talking megadoses here—up to 15,000 milligrams per day. (The recommended daily allowance is 60 milligrams.) Skeptics point out that despite several clinical trials of supplementary vitamins A, C, E, and lycopene, there is no evidence that these antioxidant pills have an effect on cancer prevention or treatment.

I do not recommend taking these pills, as some studies indicate that antioxidant supplements can interfere with radiation or chemotherapy. Further, you always take a risk by ingesting large quantities of any supplement. Instead, plan to consume antioxidants as nature intended: as part of a diet rich in colorful fruits and vegetables. For more information about food sources of antioxidants, see "Cancer Prevention: The Power Is in Your Hands" on page 218.

There is one exception to my cautionary stance on antioxidants, and that is selenium, which is discussed earlier in this chapter.

Colon Cleansing (Enemas and Colonics)

Enemas and colonics are often recommended as treatments that will help "cleanse" cancer from your body. As these treatments are both painful and dehydrating, it may come as a relief to know that there isn't a shred of evidence that they do any good. Nor is there any solid scientific reasoning for cleansing therapies.

PC-SPES

The last four letters of the herbal prostate cancer treatment PC-SPES are derived from the Latin word for "hope." In the late 1990s, this name seemed justified by a couple of promising studies. The studies showed that PC-SPES reduces the level of prostate-specific antigen (PSA), a marker for prostate cancer. It also appears to act the way estrogen does, retarding the growth of prostate cancer.

But later trials determined that even when patients showed lower levels of PSA while taking PC-SPES, their survival rates were no different from those of patients who didn't take this supplement. It seems likely that *false* hope is a serious danger of PC-SPES: by bringing down PSA levels, this treatment might lull patients and their doctors into believing that the cancer is slowing—while the tumor continues to grow undetected.

There are other reasons to avoid PC-SPES. Supposedly, it contains eight herbs: saw palmetto, ginseng, chrysanthemum, reishi mushrooms, licorice, dyer's woad, rubescens, and skullcap. But as with many other herbal mixtures, the number and kind of herbs can vary from one package to another. You never know exactly what you're getting. Worse, chemical analyses of PS-SPES have revealed contamination with traditional medications, including warfarin, an anticoagulant that can have serious health consequences if used improperly. This finding led the

FDA to issue a warning about PC-SPES in 2002. It's no longer commercially available in the United States, although people have found other avenues for sales. You may hear plenty of personal testimonies about PC-SPES, but remember that credible evidence has proven this treatment to be unhelpful and possibly dangerous.

Astragalus (Astragalus membranaceus)

Astragalus, also known as huang qi, has long been used in traditional Chinese medicine for deficiency of chi (life force). This traditional use of astragalus has led to its promotion as a tonic that can strengthen the immune systems of cancer patients.

Salespeople or alt-med advisers may tell you that studies prove the immune-boosting benefits of astragalus. It's true that a handful of Chinese trials have been performed with claims of positive results, but the scientific standards of these trials were so low that the results are difficult to assess. More and better studies are needed before we'll know if astragalus works, or even if it's safe. Until then, use caution and stay away from this herb.

Curcumin

Curcumin is a component of turmeric, a spice that flavors many Indian and rice dishes. In the laboratory, curcumin has been shown to inhibit the growth of colonic cancer cells. This finding, along with our knowledge that curcumin is poorly absorbed by the gastrointestinal tract, makes it an exciting contender as a colon-cancer therapy.

As you've seen throughout this chapter, however, it's one thing to fight cancer in a test tube and quite another to stop cancer where it counts: in people. Currently there are clinical trials under way; soon we will know whether curcumin holds up to its promising early performance.

Milk Thistle (Silybum marianum)

Milk thistle has long been used as a detoxifying herb, intended to block toxins from entering the liver and to remove any toxins that do make an appearance. Cancer patients who inquire at the health store are often told that milk thistle will regulate the immune system or protect the liver against the harmful effects of chemotherapy. Although its active ingredient, silymarin, holds promise as a powerful antioxidant, there are no good studies to support the use of milk thistle. For now, avoid this herb.

Cat's Claw (Uncaria tomentosa)

Cat's claw is popularly thought to boost the action of white blood cells and therefore support a cancer-challenged immune system. In the laboratory, cat's claw has in fact been shown to work against cancer cells. But it joins the list of other cancer treatments that remain untested in humans. Until more studies have been conducted, do not use cat's claw.

Saw palmetto, Cernilton, and Pygeum (Pygeum africanum)

Saw palmetto, Cernilton (a rye extract), and *Pygeum africanum* are all used with varying degrees of success for treatment of an enlarged prostate (see chapter 9, "Improving Prostate Health"). Each of these plant products can also slow the growth of prostate cancer cells . . . but only in the laboratory, as far as we know. Human studies of saw palmetto for prostate cancer are inconclusive, and there haven't yet been any human trials of Cernilton and *Pygeum africanum*.

Shark Cartilage

Shark cartilage is one of the most frequently used alternative therapies for cancer, and there's some logic behind its popularity. Cartilage—*any* cartilage—appears to inhibit the growth of blood vessels that are instrumental in cancer development and metastasis. This finding, combined with the intriguing fact that cartilage, unlike most other body tissues, is rarely the site of cancers, has led to profitable sales of cartilage products. (Manufacturers prefer to harvest cartilage from sharks because of their high ratio of cartilage to body weight.)

Because of the intense public interest, shark cartilage pills and powders have been put through clinical trials—where, unfortunately, they have never slowed or stopped cancer.

Mistletoe (Viscum album)

Mistletoe extract is widely used in Europe as a cancer treatment. Advocates of mistletoe and its commercial preparations (including Iscador, Helixor, and Eurixor) claim that it slows cancer growth and improves quality of life for the patient. In fact, mistletoe is the source of proteins called lectins, which inhibit cancer growth in test tubes. One of the chemicals in mistletoe, silibinin, decreases levels of prostate-specific antigen, or PSA (a marker for prostate cancer), and inhibits telomerase, one of the key enzymes involved in cancer cell growth in prostate cancer cells in the lab.

Unfortunately, these results don't transfer well from the laboratory to humans. In a 1986 study, chemotherapy combined with mistletoe extract

THE CLINIC CONUNDRUM

Dozens of alternative cancer clinics, both here in the United States and abroad, boast of their ability to cure cancer with a variety of unconventional treatments. Their claims of success, however, tend to wither when put to the test. For example, a cancer clinic in San Diego considers cancer a bacterial disease and treats patients with special diets, enemas, and vaccines. Although this clinic enjoys a strong reputation among some laypeople, a study of its technique in terminal cancer patients found no increase in survival or quality of life. Several other clinics that treat patients with combinations of drugs and other compounds have been found to produce no appreciable success. Instead of throwing your energy and money into an alternative clinic, put your resources into conventional medicine—and into alternatives that have been proven to reduce stress, fatigue, and other symptoms.

was no more effective than chemotherapy alone. Although mistletoe appeared to improve quality of life in one German study, I'm dubious of these results, because the patients knew who was receiving the mistletoe extract and who wasn't. A stronger study of 477 patients with skin cancer showed no difference in either survival rates or quality of life when mistletoe was used. In my opinion, mistletoe is best left hanging from doorways at Christmas.

The Complete Prescription for Cancer Prevention

Cardiovascular exercise: 30 minutes daily, at least 5 days a week

Diet: eat plenty of fruits and vegetables, especially yellow, orange, red, and dark green vegetables and cooked tomatoes.

Calcium: 1000 to 1500 milligrams of calcium daily from diet and supplements

Folic acid: 800 micrograms of folic acid a day from diet and supplements

The Complete Prescription for Cancer Treatment

Conventional medical therapy: as prescribed by your doctor

Diet: follow the recommendations for cancer prevention, above.

Cardiovascular exercise: as much as you reasonably perform. Try for 30 minutes daily, 5 days a week, to relieve fatigue associated with treatment.

Fish oils: one serving of fatty fish per week or 1 gram of a fish-oil supplement containing either EPA (eicosapentaenoic acid) and DHA (docosahexanoic acid)

Acupuncture: once daily for five consecutive days during chemotherapy to reduce nausea and vomiting; electroacupuncture preferred

Hypnosis: as needed to relieve cancer-related pain

Manual lymph drainage massage (for swelling associated with mastectomy and pelvic cancer surgery): as needed

Relaxation massage: as needed to relieve anxiety and possibly control pain

Group therapy/support groups: as desired to improve quality of life and reduce risk of posttraumatic stress

Mind-body therapies: as desired to reduce stress, improve sleep, and possibly control pain

Aromatherapy: as desired for relaxation and stress reduction

13

The Longevity
Top Ten

C ountless alt-med products and services promise to stop aging or even turn back the hands of time. Most are all hype and little fact, and many come with price tags that are jacked up to support the heavy costs of advertising. You can often sniff out the worst offenders by using your common sense. Shun any products or services that claim to reverse or stop aging—sorry, but that's just not possible (at least not yet). Remember that anything boasting to be a "miracle" or "fountain of youth" is probably miraculous only for the people who make a profit from the sales.

Instead, turn to my Longevity Top Ten for therapies that are proven to ward off some of the worst disorders of aging and keep your body in peak condition for as long as possible. Most of them are easy on your budget and feel great—so enjoy! I wish you a lifetime of good health.

1. CARDIOVASCULAR EXERCISE
Exercise is the number-one way to increase the pleasure you take in living and reduce your risk of heart disease, stroke, memory loss, many

cancers, diabetes, obesity, depression, anxiety, insomnia, and osteo-porosis.

You don't have to put yourself through grueling workouts to receive the benefits of cardiovascular exercise. Just find an enjoyable activity, such as walking or swimming, and push yourself just until you start breathing deeply. I advise getting a minimum of 30 minutes of cardio-vascular exercise daily for at least five days a week. If you can do more, go for it!

2. WEIGHT TRAINING

Most of us don't fear aging as much as we fear losing our independence. If you want to maintain your ability to hoist shopping bags, get yourself out of a chair, and walk up a flight of steps, start weight training *now*. In addition to beefing up your muscles, you'll also strengthen your bones and take some of the load off arthritic joints.

You don't need heavy weights or a youthful body to begin weight training. Even 80- and 90-year olds can benefit from lifting just a few pounds. To start a weight-training program, consult with a personal trainer or physical therapist. Plan to work out two or three times weekly for 15 to 20 minutes at a time.

3. THE MEDITERRANEAN AND MORE DIET

Forget multivitamins. The real power of nutrition is in food—*real* food, not pills, and definitely not the prepackaged, denatured, and flavorless stuff that so often passes for food these days. If you want to age well, eat the great-tasting foods that support healthy cell division, biochemical processes, and heart function. The best place to start is my Mediter-ranean and More Diet, outlined in detail starting on page 174. Enjoy fish, chicken, nuts, fruits, vegetables, whole grains, and even chocolate as you knock down your chances of heart disease, cancer, and dozens of other disorders that could stand between you and a long, exuberant life.

4. A GOOD NIGHT'S SLEEP

Sleep is a more potent tonic than all the supplements in the world combined. First and foremost, sleep keeps your reflexes sharp. Your life depends on those reflexes every time you drive a car, hop aboard a watercraft, or operate machinery. Just ask the former residents of Chernobyl and Three Mile Island. Investigators have linked those disasters to employee sleep loss.

Sleep does more than save your life, however. Time spent in dreamland can keep your memory fine-tuned, lift your mood, boost your levels of human growth hormone (which helps build bone and muscle mass), and keep your immune system in tiptop shape. Not to mention that you'll increase your efficiency in your daily tasks.

If you aren't getting optimal sleep, take whatever steps are necessary to put more z's in your life. You may simply need to schedule more time for sleep, just as you would schedule time to exercise or go to doctors' appointments. If you suffer from insomnia, be assured that help is available. See chapter 4, "Satisfying Sleep," for specific recommendations.

5. ENGAGEMENT WITH LIFE

If you want to stay alive, *live.* That means engaging fully with life. Start by growing a good marriage or partnership and building a strong social network of friends who can extend a hand up when you're down and who will encourage you to take care of yourself. (You can return the favor in their direction, of course.) Stay curious and challenged with work—whether paid or unpaid—that is a source of self-esteem, invigorating mental activity, and purpose. Travel, volunteer, take classes, and look for opportunities to develop new physical and intellectual skills, no matter what your age. By plunging into life's offerings, you'll feel brighter and more optimistic—which is a good thing for your health, since people with a positive attitude tend to live longer and have fewer health problems. If you maintain your social ties and stay active, you'll also be more likely to ward off Alzheimer's disease and remain independent well into old age. On the other hand, depression—which often comes with isolation and withdrawal—can increase your chances of stroke, heart problems, immune disorders, gastrointestinal problems, and even osteoporosis. Of course, you'll want to balance all this activity with calmer pursuits, so be sure to learn relaxation, meditation, or other mind-quieting techniques. They'll help you truly relish life's pleasures.

6. FOLIC ACID

Folic acid is one of the powerhouses of alternative medicine. It can prevent heart disease, reduce the risk of colon cancer, and ease depression. You need 800 micrograms of folic acid daily through diet and supplements. Good dietary sources of folic acid include fortified grain products, black-eyed peas, lentils, and cooked spinach.

7. FISH OILS (OMEGA-3 FATTY ACIDS)

Fish oils are crucial for the good health of your heart and brain—and they can even make you happier! These substances, full of omega-3 fatty acids, can improve your heart's health and reduce your risk of memory loss and Alzheimer's disease, and they appear to ease depression.

For maximum benefit, eat one to two servings of fatty fish (mackerel, herring, salmon, and tuna are good choices) a week, or take 1 gram daily of fish-oil supplements that contain EPA (eicosapentaenoic acid) and DHA (docosahexanoic acid). Do not consume more than two servings a week of fatty fish, to avoid ingesting dangerous levels of mercury and other contaminants.

8. CALCIUM

Proponents say that calcium can lower blood pressure, prevent heart disease, strengthen bones, prevent colon cancer, and reduce the symptoms of PMS . . . and they're right. Get 1000 to 1500 milligrams of calcium carbonate or calcium citrate daily from diet and supplements. Dairy products, soy products, and leafy greens are excellent sources of calcium. Be sure to get enough vitamin D as well, for proper absorption of this mineral. Read on for more information about vitamin D.

9. VITAMIN D

Without vitamin D, your body can't absorb calcium properly. This supplement is also an age-buster in its own right: it may help prevent arthritis as well as cancer of the breast, prostate, and colon.

It's a myth that most people easily get enough vitamin D through sunlight. In fact, vitamin D deficiency is a serious problem in America, especially during winter in the northern parts of the country. So get your share by exposing your skin to sunlight a few minutes several times a week, or take 1000 IU of vitamin D per day. Be sure to take no more than this, to avoid toxic reactions. For more about exposure to the sun, see "Light Therapy," below.

10. LIGHT THERAPY

You must avoid an excess of sunlight's harmful UVA and UVB rays, but don't deprive yourself of one of the most natural feel-good therapies around. A healthy dose of sunshine can improve your sleep, fight depression, relieve PMS, and help your body absorb enough vitamin D.

Everyone should get 3 to 5 minutes of sun on their exposed (no sunscreen) arms and face, two or three times each week. This will allow your skin to soak up its dose of vitamin D. Try to avoid bright, full sun while your skin is unprotected, especially if you have fair skin and burn easily.

Once you've met this requirement, it's time to slather on the sunscreen—and continue to enjoy the sunshine. This protected sun ex-

posure will help boost your mood and stimulate the production of melatonin, a hormone necessary for sleep. If that's not possible, spend as
much time as you can in a brightly lit area, preferably near a window.
When all else fails, buy a light box. Set it for at least 3000 lux (you may
need a stronger setting if you are trying to fight a particular disorder, so
see the appropriate chapter for specific recommendations) and use it for
30 minutes daily.

APPENDIX:
TAKE THIS TO YOUR DOCTOR

This appendix lists journal articles or websites that back up the recommendations in my Complete Prescriptions for each health problem. If you or your doctor would like to learn more about a particular treatment, you can look up the relevant article or articles. For those of you who don't have access to an online medical database, a librarian—especially a medical librarian—can help you track these articles down.

Chapter 2. Joint Pain: Improving Function, Easing Discomfort
GLUCOSAMINE AND CHONDROITIN SULFATE

Pavelká, Karel, Jindriska Gatterová, Marta Olejarová, Stanislav Machacek, Giampaolo Giacovelli, and Lucio C. Rovati. "Glucosamine Sulfate Use and Delay of Progression of Knee Osteoarthritis: A 3-Year, Randomized, Placebo-Controlled, Double-Blind Study." *Archives of Internal Medicine* 162, no. 18 (2002): 2113–23.

Hungerford, David S., and Lynne C. Jones. "Glucosamine and Chondroitin Sulfate Are Effective in the Management of Osteoarthritis." *Journal of Arthroplasty* 18, no. 3, Suppl 1 (2003): 5–9.

Russell, Anthony S., Ali Aghazadeh-Habashi, and Fakhreddin Jamali. "Active Ingredient Consistency of Commercially Available Glucosamine Sulfate Products." *Journal of Rheumatology* 29, no. 11 (2002): 2407–9.

TRANSCUTANEOUS ELECTRICAL NERVE STIMULATION (TENS)

Cheing, Gladys L. Y., Amy Y. Y. Tsui, Sing Kai Lo, and Christina W. Y. Hui-Chan. "Optimal Stimulation Duration of Tens in the Management of Osteoarthritic Knee Pain." *Journal of Rehabilitation Medicine* 35, no. 2 (2003): 62–68.

CAPSAICIN

Deal, Chad L., Thomas J. Schnitzer, Esther Lipstein, James R. Seibold, Randall M. Stevens, Moise D. Levy, Daniel Albert, and Frederick Renold. "Treatment of Arthritis with Topical Capsaicin: A Double-Blind Trial." *Clinical Therapeutics* 13, no. 3 (1991): 383–95.

ACUPUNCTURE

NIH Consensus Conference. "NIH Consensus Conference: Acupuncture." *JAMA* 280, no. 17 (1998): 1518–24.

AVOCADO/SOYBEAN UNSAPONIFIABLES (ASU)

Appelboom, Thierry, Joseph Schuermans, Gust Verbruggen, Yves Henrotin, and Jean Yves Reginster. "Symptoms Modifying Effect of Avocado/Soybean Unsaponifiables (Asu) in Knee Osteoarthritis: A Double Blind, Prospective, Placebo-Controlled Study." *Scandinavian Journal of Rheumatology* 30, no. 4 (2001): 242–47.

Ernst, Edzard. "Avocado-Soybean Unsaponifiables (ASU) for Osteoarthritis—a Systematic Review." *Clinical Rheumatology* 22, nos. 4–5 (2003): 285–88.

Chapter 3. Back on Track: Relief for Back and Neck Pain

CARDIOVASCULAR EXERCISE

Harris, Geoffrey R., and Jeffrey L. Susman. "Managing Musculoskeletal Complaints with Rehabilitation Therapy: Summary of the Philadelphia Panel Evidence-Based Clinical Practice Guidelines on Musculoskeletal Rehabilitation Interventions." *Journal of Family Practice* 51, no. 12 (2002): 1042–46.

Rainville, James, Carol Hartigan, Eugenio Martinez, Janet Limke, Cristin Jouve, and Mark Finno. "Exercise as a Treatment for Chronic Low-Back Pain." *Spine Journal* 4, no. 1 (2004): 106–15.

Sculco, Arthur Daniel, Donald C. Paup, Bo Fernhall, and Mario J. Sculco. "Effects of Aerobic Exercise on Low-Back Pain Patients in Treatment." *Spine Journal* 1, no. 2 (2001): 95–101.

Ylinen, Jari, Esa-Pekka Takala, Matti Nykänen, Arja Häkkinen, Esko Mälkiä, Timo Pohjolainen, Sirkka-Liisa Karppi, Hannu Kautiainen, and Olavi Airaksinen. "Active Neck Muscle Training in the Treatment of Chronic Neck Pain in Women: A Randomized Controlled Trial." *JAMA* 289, no. 19 (2003): 2509–16.

SPECIALIZED STRETCHES AND STRENGTH EXERCISES

Liddle, Sarah Dianne, G. David Baxter, and Jacqueline H. Gracey. "Exercise and Chronic Low-Back Pain: What Works?" *Pain* 107, nos. 1–2 (2004): 176–90.

WILLOW BARK

Chrubasik, Sigrun, Elon Eisenberg, Edith Balan, Tuvia Weinberger, Rachel Luzzati, and Christian Conradt. "Treatment of Low-Back Pain Exacerbations with Willow Bark Extract: A Randomized Double-Blind Study." *American Journal of Medicine* 109, no. 1 (2000): 9–14.

HYDROTHERAPY

Strauss-Blasche, Gerhard, Cem Ekmekcioglu, Gerda Vacariu, Herbert Melchart, Veronika Fialka-Moser, and Wolfgang Marktl. "Contribution of Individual Spa Therapies in the Treatment of Chronic Pain." *Clinical Journal of Pain* 18, no. 5 (2002): 302–9.

MASSAGE

Elliott, Michael A., and Lynne P. Taylor. "'Shiatsu Sympathectomy': ICA Dissection Associated with a Shiatsu Massager." *Neurology* 58, no. 8 (2002): 1302–4.

Ernst, Edzard. "Manual Therapies for Pain Control: Chiropractic and Massage." *Clinical Journal of Pain* 20, no. 1 (2004): 8–12.

PERCUTANEOUS ELECTRICAL STIMULATION (PENS)

Weiner, Debra K., Thomas E. Rudy, Ronald M. Glick, J. Robert Boston, Susan J. Lieber, Lisa A. Morrow, and Stephen Taylor. "Efficacy of Percutaneous Electrical Nerve Stimulation for the Treatment of Chronic Low-Back Pain in Older Adults." *Journal of the American Geriatrics Society* 51, no. 5 (2003): 599–608.

HEAT WRAPS

Nadler, Scott F., Deborah J. Steiner, Geetha N. Erasala, David A. Hengehold, Robert T. Hinkle, Mary Beth Goodale, Susan B. Abeln, and Kurt W. Weingand.

"Continuous Low-Level Heat Wrap Therapy Provides More Efficacy Than Ibuprofen and Acetaminophen for Acute Low-back Pain." *Spine* 27, no. 10 (2002): 1012–17.

Chapter 4. Satisfying Sleep

COGNITIVE-BEHAVIORAL THERAPY

Edinger, Jack D., William K. Wohlgemuth, Rodney A. Radtke, Gail R. Marsh, and Ruth Quillian. "Cognitive Behavioral Therapy for Treatment of Chronic Primary Insomnia: A Randomized Controlled Trial." *JAMA* 285, no. 14 (2001): 1856.

Ringold, Sarah. "Cognitive Behavior Therapy and Pharmacotherapy for Insomnia: A Randomized Controlled Trial and Direct Comparison." *JAMA* 292, no. 19 (2004): 2319.

RELAXATION TECHNIQUES

Morin, Charles M., Cheryl Colecchi, Jackie Stone, Rakesh Sood, and Douglas Brink. "Behavioral and Pharmacological Therapies for Late-Life Insomnia: A Randomized Controlled Trial." *JAMA* 281, no. 11 (1999): 991.

LIGHT THERAPY

Hood, Bernadette, Dorothy Bruck, and Gerard Kennedy. "Determinants of Sleep Quality in the Healthy Aged: The Role of Physical, Psychological, Circadian and Naturalistic Light Variables." *Age and Ageing* 33, no. 2 (2004): 159.

VALERIAN

Coxeter, P. D., P. J. Schluter, H. L. Eastwood, C. J. Nikles, and P. P. Glasziou. "Valerian Does Not Appear to Reduce Symptoms for Patients with Chronic Insomnia in General Practice Using a Series of Randomised N-of-1 Trials." *Complementary Therapies in Medicine* 11, no. 4 (2003): 215–22.

Glass, J. R., B. A. Sproule, N. Herrmann, D. Streiner, and U. E. Busto. "Acute Pharmacological Effects of Temazepam, Diphenhydramine, and Valerian in Healthy Elderly Subjects." *Journal of Clinical Psychopharmacology* 23, no. 3 (2003): 260–68.

MELATONIN

Arendt, Josephine. "Melatonin, Circadian Rhythms, and Sleep." *The New England Journal of Medicine* 343, no. 15 (2000): 1114.

Hughes, R. J., R. L. Sack, and A. J. Lewy. "The Role of Melatonin and Circadian Phase in Age-Related Sleep-Maintenance Insomnia: Assessment in a Clinical Trial of Melatonin Replacement." *Sleep* 21, no. 1 (1998): 52–68.

Almeida Montes, L. G., M. P. Ontiveros Uribe, J. Cortes Sotres, and G. Heinze Martin. "Treatment of Primary Insomnia with Melatonin: A Double-Blind, Placebo Controlled, Crossover Study." *Journal of Psychiatry and Neuroscience* 28, no. 3 (2003): 191–96.

Lushington, K., K. Pollard, L. Lack, D. J. Kennaway, and D. Dawson. "Daytime Melatonin Administration in Elderly Good and Poor Sleepers: Effects on Core Body Temperature and Sleep Latency." *Sleep* 20, no. 12 (1997): 1135–44.

Chapter 5. Taming Depression and Anxiety

COGNITIVE-BEHAVIORAL THERAPY

Doerfler, L. A., and J. A. Paraskos. "Anxiety, Posttraumatic Stress Disorder, and Depression in Patients with Coronary Heart Disease: A Practical Review for Cardiac Rehabilitation Professionals." *Journal of Cardiopulmonary Rehabilitation* 24, no. 6 (2004): 414–21.

APPLIED RELAXATION THERAPY

Ost, L. G., and E. Breitholtz. "Applied Relaxation vs. Cognitive Therapy in the Treatment of Generalized Anxiety Disorder." *Behaviour Research Therapy* 38, no. 8 (2000): 777–90.

Fisher, P. L., and R. C. Durham. "Recovery Rates in Generalized Anxiety Disorder Following Psychological Therapy: An Analysis of Clinically Significant Change in the Stai-T Across Outcome Studies since 1990." *Psychological Medicine* 29, no. 6 (1999): 1425–34.

FISH OILS

Freeman, M. P., C. Helgason, and R. A. Hill. "Selected Integrative Medicine Treatments for Depression: Considerations for Women." *Journal of the American Medical Women's Association* 59, no. 3 (2004): 216–24.

FOLATE

Jorm, A. F., H. Christensen, K. M. Griffiths, and B. Rodgers. "Effectiveness of Complementary and Self-Help Treatments for Depression." *The Medical Journal of Australia* 176 Suppl (2002): S84–96.

LIGHT THERAPY

Sher, L., J. R. Matthews, E. H. Turner, T. T. Postolache, K. S. Katz, and N. E. Rosenthal. "Early Response to Light Therapy Partially Predicts Long-Term Antidepressant Effects in Patients with Seasonal Affective Disorder." *Journal of Psychiatry and Neuroscience* 26, no. 4 (2001): 336–8.

Sumaya, I. C., B. M. Rienzi, J. F. Deegan II, and D. E. Moss. "Bright Light Treatment Decreases Depression in Institutionalized Older Adults: A Placebo-Controlled Crossover Study." *The Journals of Gerontology Series A, Biological Sciences and Medical Sciences* 56, no. 6 (2001): M356–60.

Prasko, J., J. Horacek, J. Klaschka, J. Kosova, I. Ondrackova, and J. Sipek. "Bright Light Therapy and/or Imipramine for Inpatients with Recurrent Non-Seasonal Depression." *Neuro Endocrinology Letters* 23, no. 2 (2002): 109–13.

MASSAGE

Richards, K. C., Robin Gibson, and Amy Leigh Overton-McCoy. "Effects of Massage in Acute and Critical Care." *Clinical Issues: Advanced Practices in Acute Clinical Care* 11, no. 1 (2000): 77–96.

SAINT-JOHN'S-WORT

"Effect of Hypericum Perforatum (Saint-John's-Wort) in Major Depressive Disorder: A Randomized Controlled Trial." *JAMA* 287, no. 14 (2002): 1807–14.

Fugh-Berman, A., and J. M. Cott. "Dietary Supplements and Natural Products as Psychotherapeutic Agents." *Psychosomatic Medicine* 61, no. 5 (1999): 712–28.

Markowitz, J. S., and C. L. DeVane. "The Emerging Recognition of Herb-Drug Interactions with a Focus on St. John's Wort (Hypericum Perforatum)." *Psychopharmacology Bulletin* 35, no. 1 (2001): 53–64.

Muller, W. F. "Current Saint-John's-Wort Research from Mode of Action to Clinical Efficacy." *Pharmacological Research* 47, no. 2 (2003): 101–9.

Mulrow, C. D., J. W. Williams Jr., M. Trivedi, E. Chiquette, C. Aguilar, J. E. Cornell, R. Badgett, P. H. Noel, V. Lawrence, S. Lee, M. Luther, G. Ramirez, W. S. Richardson, and K. Stamm. "Treatment of Depression—Newer Pharmacotherapies." *Evidence Report Technology Assessment* (Summ), no. 7 (1999): 1–4.

Shelton, R. C., M. B. Keller, A. Gelenberg, D. L. Dunner, R. Hirschfeld, M. E. Thase, J. Russell, R. B. Lydiard, P. Crits-Cristoph, R. Gallop, L. Todd, D. Hellerstein, P. Goodnick, G. Keitner, S. M. Stahl, and U. Halbreich. "Effectiveness of Saint-John's-Wort in Major Depression: A Randomized Controlled Trial." *JAMA* 285, no. 15 (2001): 1978–86.

Werneke, U., O. Horn, and D. M. Taylor. "How Effective Is Saint-John's-Wort?: The Evidence Revisited." *The Journal of Clinical Psychiatry* 65, no. 5 (2004): 611–17.

Wong, A. H., M. Smith, and H. S. Boon. "Herbal Remedies in Psychiatric Practice." *Archives of General Psychiatry* 55, no. 11 (1998): 1033–44.

Chapter 6. PMS: Natural Symptom Relief

CARDIOVASCULAR EXERCISE

Aganoff, J. A., and G. J. Boyle. "Aerobic Exercise, Mood States and Menstrual Cycle Symptoms." *Journal of Psychosomatic Research* 38, no. 3 (1994): 183–92.

CALCIUM

Thys-Jacobs, S., P. Starkey, D. Bernstein, and J. Tian. "Calcium Carbonate and the Premenstrual Syndrome: Effects on Premenstrual and Menstrual Symptoms. Premenstrual Syndrome Study Group." *American Journal of Obstetrics and Gynecology* 179, no. 2 (1998): 444–52.

LIGHT THERAPY

Lam, R. W., D. Carter, S. Misri, A. J. Kuan, L. N. Yatham, and A. P. Zis. "A Controlled Study of Light Therapy in Women with Late Luteal Phase Dysphoric Disorder." *Psychiatry Research* 86, no. 3 (1999): 185–92.

MAGNESIUM

Bendich, A. "The Potential for Dietary Supplements to Reduce Premenstrual Syndrome (PMS) Symptoms." *Journal of the American College of Nutrition* 19, no. 1 (2000): 3–12.

Chapter 7. Making Menopause More Comfortable

KEEPING COOL

"Treatment of Menopause-Associated Vasomotor Symptoms: Position Statement of the North American Menopause Society." *Menopause* 11, no. 1 (2004): 11–33.

CARDIOVASCULAR EXERCISE

"Treatment of Menopause-Associated Vasomotor Symptoms: Position Statement of the North American Menopause Society." *Menopause* 11, no. 1 (2004): 11–33.

PACED RESPIRATION

Freedman, R. R., and S. Woodward. "Behavioral Treatment of Menopausal Hot Flushes: Evaluation by Ambulatory Monitoring." *American Journal of Obstetrics and Gynecology* 167, no. 2 (1992): 436–39.

Freedman, R. R., S. Woodward, B. Brown, J. I. Javaid, and G. N. Pandey. "Biochemical and Thermoregulatory Effects of Behavioral Treatment for Menopausal Hot Flashes." *Menopause* 2 (1995): 211–18.

Kronenberg, Fredi, and Adriane Fugh-Berman. "Complementary and Alternative Medicine for Menopausal Symptoms: A Review of Randomized, Controlled Trials." *Annals of Internal Medicine* 137, no. 10 (2002): 805–13.

RELAXATION RESPONSE

Irvin, J. H., A. D. Domar, C. Clark, P. C. Zuttermeister, and R. Friedman. "The Effects of Relaxation Response Training on Menopausal Symptoms." *Journal of Psychosomatic Obstetrics and Gynaecology* 17, no. 4 (1996): 202–7.

SOY PRODUCTS

Tice, Jeffrey A., Bruce Ettinger, Kris Ensrud, Robert Wallace, Terri Blackwell, and Steven R. Cummings. "Phytoestrogen Supplements for the Treatment of Hot Flashes: The Isoflavone Clover Extract (ICE) Study: A Randomized Controlled Trial." *JAMA* 290, no. 2 (2003): 207–14.

Shanafelt, Tait D., Debra L. Barton, Alex A. Adjei, and Charles L. Loprinzi. "Pathophysiology and Treatment of Hot Flashes." *Mayo Clinic Proceedings* 77, no. 11 (2002): 1207–18.

van de Weijer, Peter H. M., and Ronald Barentsen. "Isoflavones from Red Clover (Promensil®) Significantly Reduce Menopausal Hot Flush Symptoms Compared with Placebo." *Maturitas* 42, no. 3 (2002): 187–93.

Upmalis, David H., Rogerio Lobo, Lynn Bradley, Michelle Warren, Frederick L. Cone, and Cathleen A. Lamia. "Vasomotor Symptom Relief by Soy Isoflavone Extract Tablets in Postmenopausal Women: A Multicenter, Double-Blind, Randomized, Placebo-Controlled Study." *Menopause* 7, no. 4 (2000): 236–42.

BLACK COHOSH

Amato, P., and D. M. Marcus. "Review of Alternative Therapies for Treatment of Menopausal Symptoms." *Climacteric* 6, no. 4 (2003): 278–84.

Kronenberg, Fredi, and Adriane Fugh-Berman. "Complementary and Alternative Medicine for Menopausal Symptoms: A Review of Randomized, Controlled Trials." *Annals of Internal Medicine* 137, no. 10 (2002): 805–13.

Wuttke, W., D. Seidlová-Wuttke, and C. Gorkow. "The Cimicifuga Preparation BNO 1055 vs. Conjugated Estrogens in a Double-Blind Placebo-Controlled Study: Effects on Menopause Symptoms and Bone Markers." *Maturitas* 44, Suppl 1 (2003): S67–77.

RED CLOVER EXTRACT

Fugh-Berman, A., and F. Kronenberg. "Red Clover (Trifolium Pratense) for Menopausal Women: Current State of Knowledge." *Menopause* 8, no. 5 (2001): 333–37.

van de Weijer, Peter H. M., and Ronald Barentsen. "Isoflavones from Red Clover (Promensil®) Significantly Reduce Menopausal Hot Flush Symptoms Compared with Placebo." *Maturitas* 42, no. 3 (2002): 187–93.

HORMONE REPLACEMENT THERAPY

Women's Health Initiative, "Women's Health Initiative Study Findings," National Institutes of Health and National Heart, Lung, and Blood Institute, http://www.whi.org/findings/.

Chapter 8. Revving Up Male Libido

EXERCISE AND WEIGHT LOSS

Bacon, C. G., M. A. Mittleman, I. Kawachi, E. Giovannucci, D. B. Glasser, and E. B. Rimm. "Sexual Function in Men Older Than 50 Years of Age: Results from the Health Professionals Follow-up Study." *Annals of Internal Medicine* 139, no. 3 (2003): 161–81.

Esposito, K., F. Giugliano, C. Di Palo, G. Giugliano, R. Marfella, F. D'Andrea, M. D'Armiento, and D. Giugliano. "Effect of Lifestyle Changes on Erectile Dysfunction in Obese Men: A Randomized Controlled Trial." *JAMA* 291, no. 24 (2004): 2978–84.

KOREAN RED GINSENG

Hong, B., Y. H. Ji, J. H. Hong, K. Y. Nam, and T. Y. Ahn. "A Double-Blind Crossover Study Evaluating the Efficacy of Korean Red Ginseng in Patients with Erectile Dysfunction: A Preliminary Report." *The Journal of Urology* 168, no. 5 (2002): 2070–73.

Chapter 9. Improving Prostate Health

SAW PALMETTO

Bent, Stephen, Christopher Kane, Katsuto Shinohara, John Neuhaus, Esther S. Hudes, Harley Goldberg, and Andrew L. Avins. "Saw Palmetto for Benign Prostatic Hyperplasia." *The New England Journal of Medicine* 354, no. 6 (2006): 557–66.

Wilt, T., A. Ishani, et al. "*Serenoa Repens* for Benign Prostatic Hypertrophy." *Cochrane Database of Systematic Reviews* 3 (2002): CD 00 1423.

ISOFLAVONE-RICH DIET

Katz, A. E. "Flavonoid and Botanical Approaches to Prostate Health." *Journal of Alternative and Complementary Medicine* 8, no. 6 (2002): 813–21.

Chapter 10. Preventing Heart Disease and Stroke

THE MEDITERRANEAN AND MORE DIET

Anderson, J. W., L. D. Allgood, A. Lawrence, L. A. Altringer, G. R. Jerdack, D. A. Hengehold, and J. G. Morel. "Cholesterol-Lowering Effects of Psyllium Intake Adjunctive to Diet Therapy in Men and Women with Hypercholesterolemia: Meta-Analysis of 8 Controlled Trials." *The American Journal of Clinical Nutrition* 71, no. 2 (2000): 472–79.

Visioli, F., and C. Galli. "Antiatherogenic Components of Olive Oil." *Current Atherosclerosis Reports* 3, no. 1 (2001): 64–67.

Zhuo, X. G., M. K. Melby, and S. Watanabe. "Soy Isoflavone Intake Lowers Serum LDL Cholesterol: A Meta-Analysis of 8 Randomized Controlled Trials in Humans." *The Journal of Nutrition* 134, no. 9 (2004): 2395–400.

CARDIOVASCULAR EXERCISE

Lee, I. M., C. H. Hennekens, K. Berger, J. E. Buring, and J. E. Manson. "Exercise and Risk of Stroke in Male Physicians." *Stroke* 30, no. 1 (1999): 1–6.

Manson, J. E., F. B. Hu, J. W. Rich-Edwards, G. A. Colditz, M. J. Stampfer, W. C. Willett, F. E. Speizer, and C. H. Hennekens. "A Prospective Study of

Walking as Compared with Vigorous Exercise in the Prevention of Coronary Heart Disease in Women." *New England Journal of Medicine* 341 (1999): 650–58.

FISH OILS

Carroll, D. N., and M. T. Roth. "Evidence for the Cardioprotective Effects of Omega-3 Fatty Acids." *The Annals of Pharmacotherapy* 36, no. 12 (2002): 1950–56.

MIND-BODY THERAPIES

Hemingway, H., and M. Marmot. "Evidence Based Cardiology: Psychosocial Factors in the Aetiology and Prognosis of Coronary Heart Disease. Systematic Review of Prospective Cohort Studies." *British Medical Journal* 318, no. 7196 (1999): 1460–67.

Linden, W., C. Stossel, and J. Maurice. "Psychosocial Interventions for Patients with Coronary Artery Disease: A Meta-Analysis." *Archives of Internal Medicine* 156, no. 7 (1996): 745–52.

MEDITATION

Canter, P. H., and E. Ernst. "Insufficient Evidence to Conclude Whether or Not Transcendental Meditation Decreases Blood Pressure: Results of a Systematic Review of Randomized Clinical Trials." *Journal of Hypertension* 22, no. 11 (2004): 2049–54.

Schneider, R. H., C. N. Alexander, F. Staggers, D. W. Orme-Johnson, M. Rainforth, J. W. Salerno, W. Sheppard, A. Castillo-Richmond, V. A. Barnes, and S. I. Nidich. "A Randomized Controlled Trial of Stress Reduction in African Americans Treated for Hypertension for over One Year." *American Journal of Hypertension* 18, no. 1 (2005): 88–98.

HAWTHORN

Chang, Q., Z. Zuo, F. Harrison, and M. S. Chow. "Hawthorn." *Journal of Clinical Pharmacology* 42, no. 6 (2002): 605–12.

De Smet, P. A. "Herbal Remedies." *New England Journal of Medicine* 347, no. 25 (2002): 2046–56.

Pittler, M. H., K. Schmidt, and E. Ernst. "Hawthorn Extract for Treating Chronic Heart Failure: Meta-Analysis of Randomized Trials." *The American Journal of Medicine* 114, no. 8 (2003): 66–74.

MAGNESIUM

Abbott, R. D., F. Ando, K. H. Masaki, K. H. Tung, B. L. Rodriguez, H. Petrovitch, K. Yano, and J. D. Curb. "Dietary Magnesium Intake and the Future Risk of Coronary Heart Disease (the Honolulu Heart Program)." *The American Journal of Cardiology* 92, no. 6 (2003): 665–69.

Al-Delaimy, W. K., E. B. Rimm, W. C. Willett, M. J. Stampfer, and F. B. Hu. "Magnesium Intake and Risk of Coronary Heart Disease Among Men." *Journal of the American College of Nutrition* 23, no. 1 (2004): 63–70.

Chapter 11. Boosting Brain Function

TAI CHI

Wolf, S. L., H. X. Barnhart, N. G. Kutner, E. McNeely, C. Coogler, and T. Xu. "Reducing Frailty and Falls in Older Persons: An Investigation of Tai Chi and Computerized Balance Training. Atlanta FICSIT Group. Frailty and Injuries: Cooperative Studies of Intervention Techniques." *Journal of the American Geriatrics Society* 44, no. 5 (1996): 489–97.

FISH OILS

Kalmijn, S., E. J. Feskens, L. J. Launer, and D. Kromhout. "Polyunsaturated Fatty Acids, Antioxidants, and Cognitive Function in Very Old Men." *American Journal of Epidemiology* 145, no. 1 (1997): 33–41.

Morris, M. C., D. A. Evans, J. L. Bienias, C. C. Tangney, D. A. Bennett, R. S. Wilson, N. Aggarwal, and J. Schneider. "Consumption of Fish and N-3 Fatty Acids and Risk of Incident Alzheimer Disease." *Archives of Neurology* 60, no. 7 (2003): 940–69.

Morris, M. C., D. A. Evans, et al. "Fish Consumption and Cognitive Decline with Age in a Large Community Study." *Archives of Neurology* 62 (2005): 1–5.

CARDIOVASCULAR EXERCISE

Churchill, J. D., R. Galvez, S. Colcombe, R. A. Swain, A. F. Kramer, and W. T. Greenough. "Exercise, Experience and the Aging Brain." *Neurobiology of Aging* 23, no. 5 (2002): 941–55.

Cotman, C. W., and N. C. Berchtold. "Exercise: A Behavioral Intervention to Enhance Brain Health and Plasticity." *Trends in Neurosciences* 25, no. 6 (2002): 295–301.

FRUITS AND VEGETABLES

Morris, M. C., D. A. Evans, J. L. Bienias, C. C. Tangney, D. A. Bennett, N. Aggarwal, R. S. Wilson, and P. A. Scherr. "Dietary Intake of Antioxidant Nutrients and the Risk of Incident Alzheimer's Disease in a Biracial Community Study." *JAMA* 287, no. 24 (2002): 3230–37.

Perkins, A. J., H. C. Hendrie, C. M. Callahan, S. Gao, F. W. Unverzagt, Y. Xu, K. S. Hall, and S. L. Hui. "Association of Antioxidants with Memory in a Multiethnic Elderly Sample Using the Third National Health and Nutrition Examination Survey." *American Journal of Epidemiology* 150, no. 1 (1999): 37–44.

NUTS AND SEEDS

Morris, M. C., D. A. Evans, J. L. Bienias, C. C. Tangney, D. A. Bennett, N. Aggarwal, R. S. Wilson, and P. A. Scherr. "Dietary Intake of Antioxidant Nutrients and the Risk of Incident Alzheimer Disease in a Biracial Community Study." *JAMA* 287, no. 24 (2002): 3230–37.

COENZYME Q$_{10}$

Muller, T., T. Buttner, A. F. Gholipour, and W. Kuhn. "Coenzyme Q$_{10}$ Supplementation Provides Mild Symptomatic Benefit in Patients with Parkinson's Disease." *Neuroscience Letters* 341, no. 3 (2003): 201–4.

Shults, C. W., D. Oakes, K. Kieburtz, M. F. Beal, R. Haas, S. Plumb, J. L. Juncos, J. Nutt, I. Shoulson, J. Carter, K. Kompoliti, J. S. Perlmutter, S. Reich, M. Stern, R. L. Watts, R. Kurlan, E. Molho, M. Harrison, and M. Lew. "Effects of Coenzyme Q$_{10}$ in Early Parkinson Disease: Evidence of Slowing of the Functional Decline." *Archives of Neurology* 59, no. 10 (2002): 1541–50.

HUPERZINE A

National Institute on Aging, Alzheimer's Disease Cooperative Study http://clinicaltrials.gov.

Chapter 12. Cancer Prevention and Treatment

CARDIOVASCULAR EXERCISE

Dimeo, F. C. "Effects of Exercise on Cancer-Related Fatigue." *Cancer* 92, no. 6 Suppl (2001): 1689–93.

DIET

National Cancer Institute, "Prevention, Genetics, Causes," National Institutes of Health, http://www.nci.nih.gov/cancertopics/prevention-genetics-causes.

ACUPUNCTURE

Shen, J., N. Wenger, J. Glaspy, R. D. Hays, P. S. Albert, C. Choi, and P. G. Shekelle. "Electroacupuncture for Control of Myeloablative Chemotherapy-Induced Emesis: A Randomized Controlled Trial." *JAMA* 284, no. 21 (2000): 2755–61.

Weiger, W. A., M. Smith, H. Boon, M. A. Richardson, T. J. Kaptchuk, and D. M. Eisenberg. "Advising Patients Who Seek Complementary and Alternative Medical Therapies for Cancer." *Annals of Internal Medicine* 137, no. 11 (2002): 889–903.

HYPNOSIS

Sellick, S. M., and C. Zaza. "Critical Review of 5 Nonpharmacologic Strategies for Managing Cancer Pain." *Cancer Prevention and Control* 2, no. 1 (1998): 7–14.

MASSAGE

Weiger, W. A., M. Smith, H. Boon, M. A. Richardson, T. J. Kaptchuk, and D. M. Eisenberg. "Advising Patients Who Seek Complementary and Alternative Medical Therapies for Cancer." *Annals of Internal Medicine* 137, no. 11 (2002): 889–903.

MIND-BODY THERAPIES

Carlson, L. E., M. Speca, K. D. Patel, and E. Goodey. "Mindfulness-Based Stress Reduction in Relation to Quality of Life, Mood, Symptoms of Stress and Levels of Cortisol, Dehydroepiandrosterone Sulfate (DHEA-S) and Melatonin in Breast and Prostate Cancer Outpatients." *Psychoneuroendocrinology* 29, no. 4 (2004): 448–74.

Ernst, E. "Complementary Therapies in Palliative Cancer Care." *Cancer* 91, no. 11 (2001): 2181–85.

FISH OILS

Hardman, W. E. "(N-3) Fatty Acids and Cancer Therapy." *The Journal of Nutrition* 134, no. 12 Suppl (2004): 3427S–30S.

AROMATHERAPY

Fellowes, D., K. Barnes, and S. Wilkinson. "Aromatherapy and Massage for Symptom Relief in Patients with Cancer." *Cochrane Database of Systematic Reviews,* no. 2 (2004): CD002287.

Louis, M., and S. D. Kowalski. "Use of Aromatherapy with Hospice Patients to Decrease Pain, Anxiety, and Depression and to Promote an Increased Sense of Well Being." *The American Journal of Hospice and Palliative Care* 19, no. 6 (2002): 381–86.

INDEX

ACE inhibitors, 172, 192
Acetaminophen, 25, 28, 54, 77, 78
Acetylcholine, 203, 210
Acetyl-N-carnitine, 213
Actos, 172
Acupuncture, 5, 10–12
    for arthritis, 12, 15, 39–40, 52, 244
    for back and neck pain, 68–70
    for cancer patients, 216, 224, 234, 256
    for depression, 112–13
    for hot flashes, 143–44
    for insomnia, 96–97
Advil, see Ibuprofen
Aerobics, 32, 62
    water, 63
Aging, 237–42
    diet and, 238
    engagement with life and, 239–40
    exercise and, 237–38
    light therapy and, 241–42
    male sexual problems and, 152
    sleep and, 80, 81, 90, 239
    supplements and, 240–41
Alcohol
    for cardiovascular health, 175–76
    sleep disturbances and, 84
    valerian and, 113
Aldomet, 131
Alendronate sodium, 150

Aleve, 28
Alpha-blockers, 153, 162–63
Alpha reductase inhibitors, 162, 164
Altace, 172
Alzheimer's disease, 199–202, 240
    alternative therapies for, 205–6, 209–14
    conventional treatments for, 203
Ambien, 86, 98
American Academy of Sleep Medicine, 94
Amodopa, 131
Androstenedione, 156
Anger management, 182, 198
Angina, 171
Angiotensin receptor blocker antagonists, 172
Antianxiety drugs, 102, 113
Anticoagulants, 147, 155
Anticonvulsants, 109
Antidepressants, 102, 106, 109–10, 113, 116
    for hot flashes, 131, 150
    for PMDD, 118–19
Antioxidants, 215
    dietary, 174, 175, 177, 183, 207–8, 219–21
    supplements, 192–93, 199, 229
Anxiety, 99–116
    chamomile tea for, 113
    cognitive-behavioral therapy for, 105
    complete prescription for, 115–16
    conventional treatments for, 102–3
    insomnia and, 99, 104

Anxiety (*cont.*)
　lifestyle changes for, 103–4
　massage for, 111
　menopause and, 134
　in PMDD, 118
　relaxation therapy for, 100, 105–6
　sources of information on treatments for,
　　247–49
　treatments to avoid for, 114–15
　valerian for, 113
　yoga for, 112
Applied relaxation therapy, 100, 105–6, 116, 247
Aricept, 203
Aristotle, 47
Arnica montana, 228
Aromatherapy, 12, 97, 226–27, 235, 257
Arteriosclerosis, 171, 177
Arthritis, 6, 14, 25–52, 204
　acupuncture for, 12, 25, 39–40
　avocado/soybean unsaponifiables for, 40–41
　capsaicin for, 25, 37–38
　complete prescription for, 52
　conventional treatments for, 28–31
　ginger for, 45–46
　glucosamine and chondroitin sulfate for, 14, 25,
　　34–37
　hydrotherapy for, 42
　magnets for, 47
　massage therapy for, 42–44
　prevention of, 31–34
　sources of information on treatments for,
　　243–44
　tai chi for, 44
　transcutaneous electrical nerve stimulation for,
　　41–42
　treatments to avoid for, 47–52
　white willow bark for, 46
　yoga for, 20, 44
Arthroscopic surgery, 30
Articulin, 48
Aspirin, 8, 29, 58, 46, 72
　for cardiovascular health, 172, 198
Astragalus, 220, 231
Avandia, 172
Avocado/soybean unsaponifiables (ASU), 40–41,
　52, 244
Ayurvedic medicine, 14, 48, 196

Back pain, 6, 53–78, 204
　acupuncture for, 68–70
　causes of, 55–56
　chiropractic manipulation for, 13, 70–71

complete prescription for controlling, 77
conventional treatments for, 57–58
exercise for, 61–65
heat wraps for, 54, 65–66
homeopathy for, 74, 75
hydrotherapy for, 66–67
magnets for, 74–76
massage for, 53, 67
osteopathy for, 71–72
percutaneous electrical nerve stimulation for,
　53, 67–68
as sign of emergency, 56–57
sources of information on treatments for, 244–46
surgery for, 59
transcutaneous electrical nerve stimulation for,
　73–74
treatments to avoid for, 76–77
white willow bark for, 53, 72–73
Balance problems, 201
　tai chi for, 206–7
　weight training for, 204
Barbiturates, 85, 86
Benadryl, 86
Benson, Herbert, 18–20, 183
Bensussen, Gale, 9
Beta blockers, 172
Beta-carotene, 193, 207, 229
Beta-sitosterol, 167
Bextra, 27, 29, 58
Biofeedback, 17, 92, 181, 182, 198
BioGest, 146
Bipolar disorder, 109
Black cohosh, 49, 129, 141–43, 150, 250–51
Black haw, 125
Blood-sugar-lowering medications, 172, 173
Blood-thinning medications, 172
Blue cohosh, 125
Bone loss, *see* Osteoporosis
Brain function, 199–214
　antioxidants for, 199, 207–8
　conventional treatments for, 202–3
　exercise and, 204
　fish oil for, 199, 205–6
　gingko biloba for, 200, 211–12
　sources of information on treatments for,
　　254–55
Breast cancer, 128, 129, 139, 141, 148, 218, 223,
　225, 226
　manual lymph node drainage after surgery for,
　　223, 235
Breast pain, 118, 122–23, 125
Bromocriptine, 118–19

Bumex, 172
Butcher's broom, 184

Caffeine, 83–84, 158, 183
Calcium, 14, 240–41
  for cancer, 222, 234
  for PMS, 117, 120–21, 125, 249
Calcium channel blockers, 172
Cancer, 3, 129, 193, 215–35
  aromatherapy and, 226–27
  back pain and, 57
  complete prescriptions for, 234
  conventional treatments for, 217–18
    (see also Chemotherapy)
  diets for, 228–29, 238
  fish oils for, 226
  group therapy and, 223
  guided imagery for, 18
  homeopathy for, 228
  HRT and risk of, 128–30
  hypnosis and, 224
  massage and, 222–23
  mind-body therapies for, 224–27
  prevention of, 218–21
  sources of information on treatments for,
    255–57
  treatments to avoid for, 229–34
  vitamins and minerals and, 106, 222
Capsaicin, 25, 37–39, 50, 52, 244
Cardiovascular exercise, 177–78, 197, 252
  for arthritis, 32, 52, 244–45
  for back and neck pain, 62, 77, 244–45
  for brain function, 204, 214, 254
  for cancer prevention and treatment, 218–19,
    221–22, 234, 255
  for depression, 103, 116
  for hot flashes, 132, 249
  for insomnia, 83, 98
  for longevity, 237–38
  for male sexual problems, 153–54, 159, 251
  for PMS, 119, 125, 249
Cardiovascular health, 169–98, 237, 238
  complete prescription for, 197–98
  coenzyme Q₁₀ for, 170, 190–91
  diet for, 170, 174–77, 238
  fish oils for, 169, 170, 179–80
  fitness and, 177–78
  garlic for, 189–90
  hawthorne for, 169, 187–88
  meditation for, 183–85
  mind-body therapies for, 181–82
  stanols and sterols for, 188–89

sources of information on treatments for,
    252–54
  tea for, 182–83
  treatments to avoid for, 191–97
  vitamins and minerals for, 169, 180–81, 185–87
Cardizem, 172
Cardura, 153
Cat's claw, 220, 232
Catapres, 131, 150
Cauda equina syndrome, 57
CDP-choline, 213–14
Celebrex, 14, 29, 58
Centers for Disease Control and Prevention, 208
Cernilton, 167–68, 232
Chamomile tea, 113
Chasteberry, 117, 122–23, 125, 129
Chelation therapy, 197
Chemotherapy, 217, 218, 226
  relief from side effects of, 216, 221–22, 224, 234
Childbirth, guided imagery for, 18
Chinese medicine, traditional, 4, 5, 21
  herbs in, 14, 45, 46, 148, 149, 231
  see also Acupuncture
Chiropractics, 13, 60, 68, 70–71, 76, 147
Chocolate, 176–77
Cholesterol, 157, 171–72
  alternative therapies for lowering, 169, 183, 186,
    188–89, 193–96
  conventional medicines for lowering, 172–73
  diet and, 174–76
  exercise and, 177
Cholestin, 194–96
Chondroitin, see Glucosamine and chondroitin
Cialis, 153, 154, 159
Cigarette smoking, 132, 218
Citicholine, 213–14
Cleansing therapies, 230
Cleopatra, 47
Clinical depression, 101, 102
Clonidine, 131, 150
Coenzyme Q₁₀, 229
  for cardiovascular health, 170, 190–91, 200
  for Parkinson's disease, 208–9, 214, 255
Cognitive-behavioral therapy (CBT), 17–18
  for cardiovascular health, 182
  for depression and anxiety, 105, 116, 247
  for insomnia, 87–90, 98, 246
  for PMS, 123–24
Cole, Scott, 207
Colon cancer, 106, 218, 220, 222, 231
Colonics, 230
Congestive heart failure, 170, 188, 190–91, 198

Coreg, 172
COX-2 inhibitors, 28–29, 58
Cozaar, 172
Cramp bark, 125
Crestor, 172, 192
Curcumin, 48, 231
Cyclosporin, 109
Cytokines, 77

Dalmane, 86
Dehydroepiandrosterone (DHEA), 156–57
Dementia, see Alzheimer's disease
Depression, 50–51, 99–116
    acupuncture for, 112–13
    aging and, 240, 241
    cognitive-behavioral therapy for, 105
    complete prescription for, 115–16
    conventional treatments for, 102–3
    fish oils for, 99, 110–11
    folic acid for, 99, 106
    in PMDD, 118
    insomnia and, 81, 99, 104
    lifestyle changes for, 103–4
    light therapy for, 99, 106–7
    massage for, 111
    menopause and, 134, 145
    Saint-John's-wort for, 99, 108–10
    sources of information on treatments for,
        247–49
    treatments to avoid for, 114–15
Devil's claw, 47–48, 76
DHA (docosahexanoic acid), 111
DHEA, 156–57, 194
Diet
    brain function and, 205–7, 214, 254–55
    cancer and, 219–21, 226, 228–29, 234, 255
    for cardiovascular health, 170, 174–77, 183, 197
    depression and, 111, 116
    menopausal symptoms and, 127, 135–41, 149,
        250
    prostate health and, 165–66
Digoxin, 109
Dihydrotestosterone (DHT), 162
Diovan, 172
Diphenhydramine, 86, 95–96
Disc degeneration, 55–56, 62
Dissolution tests, 10
Diuretics, 118, 149, 172
Doloteffin, 76
Donepezil, 203
Dong quai, 129, 148
Dopamine, 108, 115, 144

Doral, 86
Double-blind studies, see Randomized, controlled
    trials
Dysthymia, 101, 109, 116

Edecrin, 172
EDTA, 197
Effexor, 131
Egyptians, ancient, 162
Eisenberg, David, 21, 184
Electroacupuncture, 40, 143–44, 224, 234
Electroconvulsive therapy (ECT), 102–3
Endorphins, 68, 69, 103
Enemas, 230
English lavender, 97
EPA (eicosapentaenoic acid), 110
Erectile dysfunction, see Male sexual problems
Estazolam, 86
Estrogen, 128, 157
    see also Hormone replacement therapy
Eszopiclone, 86
Eurixor, 233
Evening primrose oil, 117, 124–25, 145
Evista, 131, 150
Exceptional Cancer Patient program, 224–25
Exelon, 203
Exercise
    for arthritis, 30, 32, 52
    for back and neck pain, 61–65
    see also Cardiovascular exercise; Weight training

Fiber, 174
Fibromyalgia, 51
Finasteride, 162, 164
Fish oils, 240
    for brain function, 199, 205–6, 214, 254
    for cancer, 226, 234
    for cardiovascular health, 169, 170, 174, 175,
        197, 252
    for depression, 99, 110–11, 116, 247
5-HTP, 114–15
Flavonoids, 175, 177, 192
Flomax, 163
Fluoxetine, 131
Flurazepam, 86
Folic acid/folate, 240
    for cancer, 222, 234
    for cardiovascular health, 169, 180–81, 197
    for depression, 99, 106, 116, 247
Food and Drug Administration (FDA), 8, 27, 29,
        137, 158, 190, 195, 231
Fosamax, 150

GABA, 108
Galantamine, 203
Galen, 46
Garlic, 189
Gate-control theory, 73
Generalized anxiety disorder (GAD), 100, 102
German Ministry of Health, Kommission E, 8, 95,
   97, 122, 212
Ginger, 45–46
Gingko biloba, 157, 184, 198, 200, 202, 211–12
Ginseng, 147–48
   for male sexual problems, 154–55, 159, 251–52
Glucophage, 172
Glucosamine and chondroitin sulfate, 14, 25,
   34–37, 52, 243
Glucotrol, 172
Glutamate, 203
Glyceryl-trinitrate (GTN), 38
Greeks, ancient, 144
Group therapy, 223, 235
Guaiacum resin, 49
Guggulipid, 196
Guided imagery, 18, 92, 133, 227

Hahnemann, Samuel, 15
Hand-eye coordination, 201
Hawthorn, 169, 187–88, 198, 253
Health Professionals Study, 153–54, 178
Heart disease
   clinical depression and, 101
   COX-2 inhibitors and, 29, 58
   erectile dysfunction drugs and, 153
   folic acid and, 106
   HRT and, 129
   observational studies of, 3
   phytoestrogens and, 135, 137–38
   prevention of, see Cardiovascular health
   SERMs and, 130
   yohimbe and, 158
HeartCare, 188, 198
Heat wraps, 54, 65–66, 77, 245–46
Helixor, 233
Herbs, 13–14
   for arthritis, 26
   for menopause, 132
   psychiatric medications and, 105
   see also specific herbs
Herniated discs, 55–56, 62
High blood pressure, 171–72
   conventional medications for, 172–73
   erectile dysfunction drugs and, 153
   exercise for, 178

fish oils for, 169, 179
garlic and, 189
meditation for, 184–85
yohimbe and, 158
Hip fractures, 201
Hip replacement surgery, 31
Hippocrates, 144
HIV, 109, 218
Homeopathy, 10, 15–16
   for back pain, 74, 75
   for cancer, 228
   for menopause, 146
   for PMS, 124
Homocysteine, 180–81
Honolulu Heart Study, 185
Hormone replacement therapy (HRT), 127–32,
   139, 142, 150, 203, 251
Hot flashes, 128–31, 133
   acupuncture for, 143–44
   herbs for, 141, 142, 144–46
   complete prescription for, 149–50
   paced respiration for, 128, 133, 134
   phytoestrogens for, 135–36, 140
   relaxation response for, 133–35
   simple steps for relieving, 132
   sources of information on treatments for,
      249–51
   treatments to avoid for, 147
Huang qi, 220, 231
Human growth hormone (HGH), 81, 239
Huperzine A, 9, 200, 209–10, 214, 255
Hyaluronic acid, 29
Hydrochlorothiazide, 172
Hydrotherapy, 16
   for arthritis, 6, 42, 52
   for back and neck pain, 56, 66–67, 77, 78
   for insomnia, 94–95, 98
   sources of information on, 245
Hygroton, 172
Hypnosis, 133, 224, 225, 235, 256
Hytrin, 153, 163

Ibuprofen, 27–29, 45, 52
Impotence, see Male sexual problems
Incontinence, 57
Inderal, 172
India, traditional medicine in, see Ayurvedic
   medicine
Insomnia, 17, 18, 79–98
   acupuncture for, 96–97
   anxiety and, 99, 104
   aromatherapy for, 97

Insomnia (*cont.*)
   arthritis and, 28
   cognitive-behavioral therapy for, 87–90
   complete prescription for, 98
   conventional treatments for, 85–87
   depression and, 99, 101, 104
   hydrotherapy for, 94–95
   light therapy for, 79, 90–91, 241–42
   melatonin for, 79, 92–94
   menopause and, 128, 129, 135, 141, 142, 145
   in PMDD, 118
   relaxation therapies for, 91–92
   sources of information on treatments for,
      246–47
   treatments to avoid for, 97–98
   valerian for, 80, 95–96
Institute of Medicine, Food and Nutrition, 123
Insulin, 172
Integrative medicine, 7
Iscador, 233
Isocarboxazid, 148, 155
Isoflavones, 136–41, 150, 165–66, 168, 252

Joint pain, *see* Arthritis
Kava kava, 97–98, 114, 149
Knee replacement surgery, 31

Laboratory studies, 5
Laetrile, 216–17
L-arginine, 155–56, 191–92
Lasix, 172
Lavender, 97
Leaf, Alexander, 1
Levitra, 153, 154, 159
Lexapro, 102
L-glutamate, 108
Licorice, 149
Lidocaine, 38
Light therapy, 241–42
   for depression, 99, 106–7, 116, 248
   for insomnia, 79, 90–92, 98, 246
   for PMDD, 121, 125, 249
Lipitor, 172, 192
Local acupuncture, 70
Longevity, 237–42
Lopressor, 172
Lotensin, 172
L-tryptophan, 114–15
Lunesta, 86, 98
Lutein, 192
Lycopene, 192, 229

MacArthur Foundation Study of Successful
   Aging, 204
Macrobiotic diets, 228
Magnesium, 121–22, 125, 185–86, 198, 249, 253–54
Magnets, 47, 74–76
Male sexual problems, 151–59
   complete prescription for, 159
   conventional treatments for, 151–53
   ginseng for, 151, 154–55
   L-arginine for, 152, 155–56
   after prostate surgery, 163
   sources of information on treatments for,
      251–52
   treatments to avoid for, 156–58
   weight and, 153–54
Manual lymph node drainage, 223, 235
Marplan, 148, 155
Massage, 6, 10, 16–17
   for arthritis, 6, 42–44, 52
   for back and neck pain, 60, 67, 245
   for cancer patients, 222–23, 227, 235, 256
   for depression and anxiety, 111, 116, 248
McQueen, Steve, 216
Meditation, 18–19, 92, 182–85, 198, 225, 226, 253
Mediterranean and More Diet, 170, 171, 174–77,
   197, 238, 252
Melatonin, 79, 90, 92–94, 98, 242, 246–47
Memantine, 203
Memory loss, 135, 199, 200
   countering, 205, 237, 239, 240
   insomnia and, 81
   major, *see* Alzheimer's disease
   phytoestrogens and, 138
Menopause, 119, 127–50, 157
   black cohosh for, 141–43
   complete prescription for, 149–50
   conventional treatments for, 127, 129–31
   homeopathy for, 146
   phytoestrogens for, 127, 135–41
   sleep disturbances and, 80
   sources of information on treatments for,
      249–51
   treatments to avoid for, 147–49
   wild Mexican yam for, 127, 145–46
   see also Hot flashes
Metastatic cancer, 217
Methyldopa, 131
Mevacor, 172, 192, 193
Micronase, 172
Migraines, 51
Mild cognitive impairment (MCI), 202, 209–10, 214

Milk thistle, 220, 231–32
Mind-body therapies, 17–20
    for cancer patients, 224–26, 235, 256
    for heart-attack treatment and prevention,
        181–82, 198, 253
    see also specific therapies
Minipress, 153
Mistletoe, 215, 220, 233–34
Mobilization therapy, 13
Monoamine oxidase inhibitors (MAOIs), 148, 155
Monopril, 172
Monounsaturated fats, 174, 175
Mood changes
    in menopause, 128, 130, 141, 142, 145
    see also Depression
Motrin, see Ibuprofen
MSM (Methylsulfonylmethane), 48–49
Multiprocessing skills, 200–201
Muscle relaxants, 58
Muscle weakness, back pain with, 56

Namenda, 203
Naprosyn, 28
Naproxen, 28
Nardil, 148, 155
National Center for Complementary and
    Alternative Medicine, 3, 7
National Cholesterol Education Programs, 188
National Health and Nutrition Examination
    Survey, 208
National Institute on Aging, 103, 210
National Institutes of Health (NIH), 39, 68–69,
    96–97, 209, 216–17
Native Americans, 49, 50, 137, 141, 164
Naturetin, 172
Neck pain, 53–78
    acupuncture for, 68–70
    causes of, 55–56
    complete prescription for controlling, 77–78
    exercise for, 61–65
    heat wraps for, 54, 65–66
    homeopathy for, 74, 75
    hydrotherapy for, 66–67
    massage for, 53
    osteopathy for, 71–72
    as sign of emergency, 57
    surgery for, 59
    transcutaneous electrical nerve stimulation for,
        73–74
    treatments to avoid for, 76–77
Neurotransmitters, 102, 108, 115, 122, 191

Niacin, 186–87
Nitric oxide, 191–92
Nitroglycerin, 153
Nonsteroidal anti-inflammatory drugs (NSAIDs),
    72–73
    for arthritis, 28, 29, 41, 46, 48, 51, 52
    for back and neck pain, 58, 77, 78
    for PMS, 118
Norepinephrine, 102, 108
Norvasc, 172
Numbness, back or neck pain with, 56–57
Nurses' Health Study, 178
Nutritional Prevention of Cancer Study, 219

Observational studies, 3–4
Omega-3 fatty acids, 117, 124
    see also Fish oils
Oral contraceptives, 109, 118, 144
Osteoarthritis, see Arthritis
Osteopathy, 71–72
Osteoporosis, 129, 131, 150
    back pain and, 57
    phytoestrogens for, 135, 138–39

Paced respiration, 128, 133, 134, 149
Parkinson's disease, 50, 115, 200, 202
    coenzyme Q_{10} for, 208–9, 214
    conventional treatments for, 203
Parnate, 148, 155
Paroxetine, 131
Pauling, Linus, 229
Paxil, 108, 131
PC-SPES, 230–31
Percutaneous electrical nerve stimulation (PENS),
    53, 64, 67–68, 74, 77, 245
Peripheral vascular disease, 184, 186, 198
Permixon, 164
Peyronie's disease, 213
Phenelzine, 148, 155
Phosphatidylserine (PS), 212
Physical therapy, 17, 30, 41–42
    for back and neck pain, 63–64, 77, 78
Phytochemicals, 162, 164, 167
Phytoestrogens, 135–41
    see also Soy products
PMS, 14, 117–25, 241
    calcium for, 117, 120–21
    cardiovascular exercise for, 119
    chasteberry for, 117, 122–23
    cognitive-behavioral therapy for, 123–24
    complete prescription for, 125

PMS (*cont.*)
    conventional medicine for, 118–19
    homeopathy for, 124
    light therapy for, 121
    magnesium for, 121–22
    treatments to avoid for, 124–25
    vitamin B_6 for, 117, 123
Pollen extracts, 167–68
Pravachol, 172, 192
Precose, 172
Premenstrual dysphoric disorder (PMDD), 118–19, 121
Premenstrual syndrome, *see* PMS
Priapism, 153
Procardia, 172
Progesterone, 127, 128, 145
    see also Hormone replacement therapy
Progressive muscle relaxation, 91
Promensil, 141, 150
Proscar, 162, 164
ProSom, 86
Prostate cancer, 129, 157, 162, 165, 215, 219, 225, 230–31, 233
Prostate enlargement, 14, 161–68
    beta-sitosterol for, 167
    complete prescription for, 168
    conventional treatments for, 162–63
    isoflavones for, 165–66
    plant-based foods for, 161
    pygeum for, 166–67, 232
    saw palmetto for, 161, 164–65, 232
    sources of information on treatments for, 252
    treatments to avoid for, 167–68
Prozac, 108, 131
Psychoanalysis, 102
Pygeum, 166, 167, 232

Quazepam, 86

Radiation therapy, 217, 218, 221–22
Raloxifene, 131, 150
Ramelteon, 86, 98
Randomized, controlled trials (RCTs), 3–4, 6, 13
Red clover, 135–40, 150, 166, 251
Red yeast rice extract, 169, 194–96
Relaxation therapies, 18–20
    for anxiety, 100, 105–6, 116
    for cancer patients, 225, 226
    for cardiovascular health, 171, 182, 198
    for hot flashes, 133–35, 149, 250
    for insomnia, 83, 91–92, 98, 246
Remifemin, 142, 143, 150

Reminyl, 203
Restoril, 95–96
Reumalex, 49
Rivastigmine, 203
Rolfing, 44, 57
Romans, ancient, 16, 46
Rozerem, 86, 98

S-adenosyl-L-methionine, 106
Saint-John's-wort, 99, 108–10, 116, 248–49
SAMe (S-adenosyl-L-methionine), 50–52, 115
SARMs (selective androgen receptor modulators), 158
Sarsparilla, 49
Saw palmetto, 14, 161, 164–65, 167, 168, 220, 232, 252
Sciatica, 58
Selective serotonin reuptake inhibitors (SSRIs), 102, 108, 109
Selenium, 192, 193, 219, 229–30
SERM (selective estrogen receptor modulators), 130
Serotonin, 102, 106, 108, 109, 115, 122
Shark cartilage, 215, 232–33
Shiatsu, 44, 57, 245
Shiitake mushrooms, 220, 228–29
Siegel, Bernie, 224–25
Situational depression, 100–101, 103
Sleep, 239
    disturbances of, *see* Insomnia
Small, Gary, 205
Smoking, 132, 218
Social ties, maintaining, 239–40
Sonata, 85, 98
Soy products
    for cardiovascular health, 176
    for menopausal symptoms, 127, 135–41, 149, 250
    for prostate health, 165–66
Stanols, 188–89
Statins, 172, 192–93, 203
Steroid injections, 29, 58
Sterols, 188–89
Stimulus control, 88
Stinging nettle, 49–50
Strength training, *see* Weight training
Stress
    insomnia and, 87, 98
    mind-body therapies for, 17–20, 182, 198
    yoga for, 21
    see also Anxiety
Stroke, 129
    prevention of, *see* Cardiovascular health

Substance P, 25, 37
Sunlight, exposure to, 103–4
    see also Light therapy
Supplements, 7–11, 13–14, 51
    certification of, 9
    dissolution tests on, 10
    psychiatric medications and, 105
    where to buy, 9–10
    see also specific supplements
Support groups, 223, 235
Surgery
    for back and neck pain, 54, 59
    for cancer, 217, 223
    for joint pain, 29–31
    for prostate enlargement, 162, 163, 168

Tai chi, 20, 214
    for arthritis, 6, 44, 52
    for balance, 206–7, 254
Tamsulosin hydrochloride, 163
Tea, 177, 182–83
Tenormin, 172
Terazosin hydrochloride, 163
Testosterone, 128, 129, 152, 157–58, 162, 164
Theophylline, 109
Tocotrienols, 192, 193
Transcutaneous electrical nerve stimulation
        (TENS), 67, 244
    for arthritis, 41–42, 52
    for back and neck pain, 73–74
Transient ischemic attacks, 171
Tranylcypromine, 148, 155
Triglycerides, 176, 178, 195
Triptans, 109
Tylenol, 25, 28
Tyramine, 158

U.S. Pharmacopeia, 164
Ubiquinon, 190

Vaginal dryness, 128, 131, 150
Valerian, 80, 95–96, 98, 113, 246
Vasotec, 172

Venlafaxine, 131
Veramil, 172
Viagra, 152–55, 159
Vinpocetine, 213
Vioxx, 27, 29, 58
Visualization, 18
    see also Guided imagery
Vitamin A, 229
Vitamin B_6, 117, 123
Vitamin B_{12}, 180–81
Vitamin C, 33, 34, 192, 207, 229
Vitamin D, 33–34, 120–21, 125, 222, 241
Vitamin E, 41, 146, 192, 193, 207–8, 229

Warfarin, 109
Water aerobics, 63
Weight loss
    for arthritis prevention, 32
    for male sexual problems, 153–54, 159, 251
Weight training
    for arthritis, 30, 32, 52
    for back and neck pain, 64–65, 67, 245
    for balance, 204, 214
    bone density and, 131, 139, 149
    for longevity, 238
Wild yam, 125, 127, 145–46
Willow bark, 26, 46, 49, 53, 245
Women's Health Initiative (WHI), 129–30,
        203

Yoga, 20–21
    for anxiety, 112, 116
    for arthritis, 6, 44, 52
    for cancer patients, 225, 226
Yohimbe, 143, 158

Zaleplon, 85
Zestril, 172
Zinc, 48
Zocor, 172, 192
Zoloft, 108, 109, 118
Zolpidem, 86
Zostrix, 39

ABOUT THE AUTHORS

Edward L. Schneider, M.D., is one of the nation's preeminent experts on longevity. He is known for his work in the landmark MacArthur Foundation Study of Successful Aging and was deputy director of the National Institute on Aging. Dr. Schneider was the executive director of the Ethel Perry Andrus Gerontology Center and the dean of the Leonard Davis School of Gerontology at the University of Southern California in Los Angeles, where he is currently dean emeritus. He also delivers lectures about health and longevity worldwide. He lives in Los Angeles with his wife and four children.

Leigh Ann Hirschman lives in Indiana with her husband and two young daughters.